# EVA FRASER'S
# FACIAL WORKOUT

PENGUIN BOOKS

PENGUIN BOOKS

UK | USA | Canada | Ireland | Australia
India | New Zealand | South Africa

Penguin Books is part of the Penguin Random House group of companies
whose addresses can be found at global.penguinrandomhouse.com.

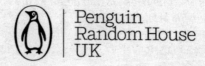

Penguin
Random House
UK

First published by Viking 1991
Published in Penguin Books 1992
Re-issued in this edition 2017
001

Copyright © Eva Fraser, 1991
Illustrations copyright © Debbie Hinks, 1991

The moral right of the author has been asserted

Printed in Great Britain by Clays Ltd, St Ives plc

A CIP catalogue record for this book is available from the British Library

ISBN: 978-1-405-93308-7

www.greenpenguin.co.uk

PENGUIN BOOKS

# EVA FRASER'S FACIAL WORKOUT

Born in England in 1928, Eva Fraser grew up to be keenly interested in sport, and her first job was working as a tennis and squash instructor. She then went to work for one of London's top photographers, soon becoming involved in the more technical side of photographic printing.

She travelled widely, establishing a career in tapestry restoration until a chance meeting in 1978 with Eva Hoffman. Madame Hoffman, then 76 years old, trained Eva in her facial exercise techniques, which she had devised with a doctor colleague in the 1930s. On her retirement Madame Hoffman encouraged Eva to take over her work.

This method is taught in London in private one-to-one sessions. Through books and DVDs it is now available to a wider audience.

www.evafraser.com

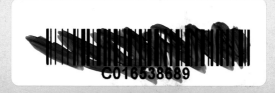

C016538689

# CONTENTS

CONTENTS

# ACKNOWLEDGEMENTS

My special thanks to my friends and colleagues for their help and support: my partner Marion; my solicitor, Anne Harrison, of Harbottle and Lewis, for all her expert advice; Christine Pearce, a PA supreme; Gary Williams, for his excellent photographs; and Kathryn Marsden for her invaluable advice on vitamins and minerals.

# INTRODUCTION

In recent years, keeping fit has become more and more popular – and quite rightly so. Keeping our bodies strong and fit should be the concern of us all. But – leaving aside plastic surgery, creams and potions – where does the face fit into all this?

Many people I meet are quite unaware of the structure of the face, even to the extent of not realizing that we have any facial muscles at all. But if we didn't have them, how would we blink? How would we smile? How would we grimace? We do all these through the use of facial muscles.

Many of the facial muscles are hardly used at all, though – except, perhaps, to frown or to squint. These bad habits can all be changed, however, and the muscles can be retrained to work correctly, gradually reversing the signs of ageing.

I don't believe in eternal youth, other than in spirit. However, we can all do an enormous amount towards staying younger and fitter in mind and body. The confidence and well-being this brings about are remarkable.

The muscles of the face differ from those of the body in that they are attached directly to the skin that covers them. This means that when the facial muscles sag, the skin attached to them sags too. In fact the slackening of the facial muscles is one of the main causes of the sagging and drooping that most of us eventually experience, leading to bags under the eyes, loose folds of skin on the upper eyelids, pouches, jowls, turkey-necks . . . Need I go on? If the body were as neglected as so many faces appear to be, some of us would have muscles so wasted away that we would barely be able to walk.

Why do we neglect our facial muscles so much, perhaps just pinning our hopes on yet another miracle cream? Many creams can improve the texture of the skin, of course, but so far there is no cream that can improve the tone and strength of a muscle. If your stomach muscles are slack, all the creams in the world will do nothing to tighten them, and it is the same with the face. Muscles have to be exercised in order to become firm and fit!

The methods I have outlined in this book are not new. In 1978 I was fortunate to meet a very impressive woman by the name of Eva Hoffman. Way back in 1930, with the assistance of a doctor, she had devised a method of exercising the facial muscles. She spent the following years travelling the world giving private lessons in her technique to a rather wealthy clientele. When we met, Eva was seventy-six, but looked as if she was in her fifties. She was just amazing. And her secret was simply facial exercises. At that time Eva had been retired for six years, but, after some persuasion, she gave me her course, and later trained me to carry on her work. Since then I have modified some of her techniques considerably, but her basic approach has remained the same.

My gratitude to Eva has no bounds, not only for the peace of mind she gave me (now, at the age of sixty-two, I have no fear of ageing), but also on behalf of the countless others who have benefited from her methods.

This book is therefore dedicated to Eva Hoffman.

# EXPLANATION

The aim of this book is to improve the facial contour – naturally. There is an enormous amount you can do for yourself to delay the inevitable ageing process. Exercise is undoubtedly one of the chief factors in staying more youthful and confident at whatever age, and the good news is that it's never too late to start!

Of course, the earlier you start to look after yourself the better, but I have known people at seventy and eighty who have found a great improvement in their well-being and appearance following the Facial Workout programme.

A question I am sometimes asked is, 'Isn't this all rather vain? I would feel guilty spending so much time on myself.' But how can exercising and keeping fit be vain? Looking after yourself means that, as you get older, you are more likely to stay strong and fit and able to help others. Also, the time spent on this programme is minimal. At first you will obviously have to learn the exercises, and this takes a certain amount of concentration and time. But over the weeks the exercises will become easier, and ten minutes a day is then enough to keep your face toned and fit.

Your Facial Workout exercises are in the first part of this book. They are divided into five Workout programmes, starting with a simple Basic routine and progressing gradually to the Advanced and final stage.

At the start of each programme you will find a 'Programme Planner'. Read this carefully, to make your progress more efficient and less time-consuming.

You may feel tempted to rush through the exercises, feeling that the more you do, the quicker will be the results. In fact the reverse is true – a regular, steady pace will give you the best results by far.

Before you start the first Workout programme, though, read the background information on the next couple of pages, so that you approach the exercises as well-prepared as possible.

## THE MUSCLES OF YOUR FACE

Before starting the Basic Workout programme, have a look at the muscle chart opposite.

You may not have been aware that we all have this amazing muscle structure under our skin. There is no need to learn the names of the various muscles that we will be working on, but, if you were not aware of them before, you should now appreciate how lack of use and improper working of these muscles can cause the face to age much sooner than it need, just like a badly exercised body.

It is not so much lines on the face that give the appearance of age, unless they are very pronounced, but the drooping and sagging of the facial muscles. The result can be very depressing to many people.

If you follow this Facial Workout course as instructed, you will feel a definite improvement in your muscle tone in just a few weeks – your face will have lost that 'melting wax' feeling that you may experience at times.

When you reach the Advanced Workout programme you will not only feel an improvement but also *see* your face gradually 'lifting' – your upper cheeks will become plumper, any folds on your upper eyelids will decrease, the corners of your mouth will become firmer and any lines on your upper lip will be reduced. Your neck and jaw line will become firmer, and any jowls will gradually lessen and eventually disappear. In fact there will be a general all-over improvement.

The neck and jaw line can sometimes take longer than the rest of the face to show an improvement – it very much depends on the extent to which your muscles have deteriorated. However, do keep going.

It is unlikely that this course will make you look younger than your daughter – if you have one – but, at whatever age you start, you will see and feel an immense improvement. You will certainly feel more confident and look younger than you do now.

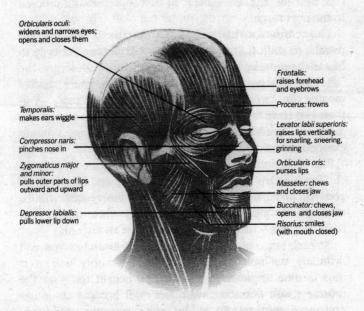

Orbicularis oculi:
widens and narrows eyes;
opens and closes them

Frontalis:
raises forehead
and eyebrows

Procerus: frowns

Temporalis:
makes ears wiggle

Levator labii superioris:
raises lips vertically,
for snarling, sneering,
grinning

Compressor naris:
pinches nose in

Orbicularis oris:
purses lips

Zygomaticus major
and minor:
pulls outer parts of lips
outward and upward

Masseter: chews
and closes jaw

Buccinator: chews,
opens  and closes jaw

Depressor labialis:
pulls lower lip down

Risorius: smiles
(with mouth closed)

# HOW TO USE THIS BOOK FOR
# MAXIMUM RESULTS

The first part of this book contains all your Facial Workout routines.

Let me explain.

Your Facial Workouts are divided into five separate programmes.

It is important that you keep to the Basic Workout routine until you are absolutely sure that you know it thoroughly and can carry out the Basic Workouts with ease and effect. Then – *and only then* – you should proceed to the next stage.

The reason for this is that the muscles of the face are usually so unfit that at first it takes a little time not only to locate the muscles but also to move them. Don't forget, the facial muscles have possibly just been 'sitting there', barely moving for twenty, thirty or forty years or more. You therefore have to get these muscles used to movement and discipline, gradually leading up to the advanced lifting exercises in the final Workouts.

The programmes are structured so that your facial muscles are built up and strengthen gradually and effectively. If you try to rush through the course, the results will be minimal. So please really concentrate while doing your daily routines – you are not competing with anyone!

At each stage of the five Workout programmes you will definitely see and feel a difference. Not only will your muscle tone improve: your skin will benefit too – as the muscle tissue develops, your face will become smoother and more youthful. So do put aside some time for yourself each day. Relax and concentrate – the results will be amazing!

Further on in the book I have included sections on make-up, hair and clothes which you may find useful.

Among the many people I meet every day I find that some look infinitely more attractive without make-up or with a minimal amount. But there are others who are completely transformed by make-up – they simply glow!

The same applies to clothes. We all have clothes that give us confidence, particular outfits that we just feel 'good' in. But other clothes seem to do nothing for us. The reason for this is mainly the colours and shapes we choose, so it is important to be aware of this. Study the clothes that do something for you and those that don't. It certainly makes shopping easier to have this awareness, and the tips I will mention later can help to give a more youthful appearance.

I have also included a section on body Workouts. You may have your own fitness routines, but if you need a few limbering-up exercises you will find that those given later are effective and quick to do. You might consider joining a keep-fit class, but this section will in any case give you a good basic fitness programme.

There are also sections on diet and – most important – knowing your vitamins and minerals for health.

Various methods of facial massage are included, which are excellent for the skin and for the general tone of the underlying tissue. But these are not conventional methods of massage for the face, as you will see.

At the start of each of the five Workout programmes you will find a simple explanation in the form of a 'Programme Planner'. Follow this and you can't go wrong.

Please try to resist flicking through this book, trying out the facial exercises at random. You would find them difficult and ineffective, possibly causing you to give up before you've even started.

So, start at the beginning and take your time – the results will be really worthwhile!

# WARMING UP BEFORE YOU START

Before your start your exercise programme, try to relax. Choose a time when you have space for yourself. We are all busy, but we all find time for the things we want to do. Set aside this time just for you, and don't let yourself be distracted.

Sit quietly, close your eyes and let go.

Feel the tension leave your head, brow, eyes, cheeks, mouth, jaw, neck, shoulders, chest, arms, torso, legs.

Breathe in deeply, then breathe out – feeling at peace with yourself.

Relax like this for one to two minutes, or longer if you wish.

Then start to warm up with the following neck movements.

# NECK EXERCISE 1

The neck is part of the spinal column, and tension can be a problem in this area. This exercise and those that follow can help to relieve some of this tension.

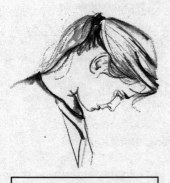

1  Sit or stand. Your spine should be straight but relaxed. Breathe in and breathe out slowly.

2  Gently lower your head forward until your chin rests on or near your chest. You will feel a gentle stretch at the back of your neck. Slowly breathe in and breathe out.

*Don't use any force when doing these movements.*

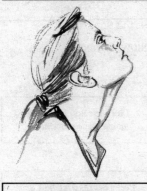

3  Now slowly raise your head and lower it backwards towards your shoulder-blades. Relax in this position. Stretch your chin upwards. Breathe in and breathe out.

4  Raise your head again, slowly.

Do this three times.

*Make relaxed, smooth movements. Keep your jaw relaxed.*

## *NECK EXERCISE 2*

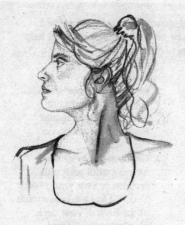

1 Sit or stand. Your spine should be straight but relaxed. Breathe in and breathe out slowly.

2 With your head and neck erect, turn your head slowly to the right. Count to five.

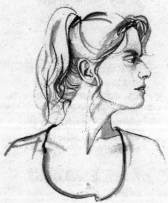

3 Now turn your head slowly to the left. Count to five.

Do this three times.

> *Don't use any force when doing these movements.*

> *Feel a gentle stretch in your neck when your head is turned. Keep your jaw relaxed.*

## NECK EXERCISE 3

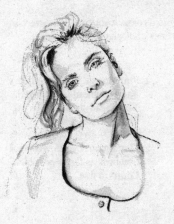

1 Sit or stand. Your spine should be straight but relaxed. Breathe in and breathe out slowly.

2 With your head and neck erect, lower your head to the right, bringing your right ear towards your right shoulder.
Count to five.

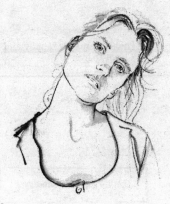

3 Raise your head slowly, then lower it to the left, bringing your left ear towards your left shoulder.
Count to five.

Do this three times.

---

*Don't force your head down towards your shoulders.*

---

*Let the weight of your head govern the distance you go.*

# EYE EXERCISE 1

Eye exercises are a vital part of your Workout routine. This exercise and the two that follow are easy and take very little time.

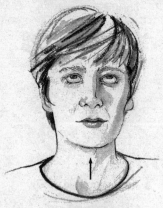

1 Stand or sit. Your shoulders and jaw should be relaxed. Your head should be facing forward and erect.

2 Moving only your eyes, look upwards as far as possible. Count to five.

3 Lower your eyes rapidly and look down.
Count to five.

Do this three times.

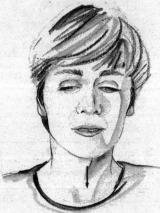

*Don't tense your shoulders or jaw.*

*Keep your head still. Move only your eyes. Breathe steadily.*

## *EYE EXERCISE 2*

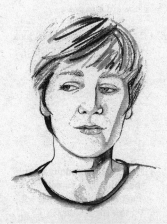

1 Stand or sit. Your shoulders and jaw should be relaxed. Your head should be facing forward and erect.

2 Look to the right, moving your eyes only.
  Count to five.

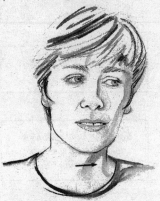

3 Rapidly look to the left – eyes only.
  Count to five.

Do this three times.

---

*Don't tense your shoulders or jaw.*

---

*Keep your head still. Move only your eyes. Breathe steadily.*

---

## EYE EXERCISE 3

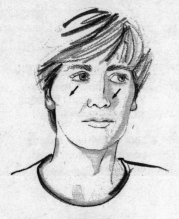

1 Stand or sit. Your shoulders and jaw should be relaxed. Your head should be facing forward and erect.

2 Moving only your eyes, look diagonally up to the left, then rapidly diagonally down to the right. Do this three times.

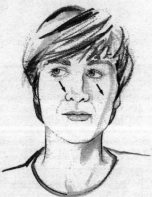

3 Now look diagonally up to the right, then rapidly diagonally down to the left. Do this three times.

Do this three times.

> *Don't tense your shoulders or jaw.*

> *Keep your head still. Move only your eyes. Breathe steadily.*

When you have completed these exercises, close your eyes and relax your brow, eyes, facial muscles, neck and shoulders, etc. Sit quietly in the relaxed state for a moment or two. Breathe in and breathe out.

# THE BASIC WORKOUT

## PROGRAMME PLANNER

The neck and eye warm-up exercises (pages 9–14) should
be performed daily, at any time.

### THE BASIC WORKOUT

Time of day:    Any time (except when tired)
Time needed:   At first – about five minutes, twice a day
                 Later – about two minutes, twice a day

*Sit in front of a mirror.*

Start with one to two minutes of basic neck and eye warm-up exercises.

Then follow the Basic Workout programme (pages 16–22).

When you are familiar with this programme you can (if you like) continue your daily workout without a mirror, sitting, standing, lying down – even in bed. But at first you *must* be in front of a mirror, as you must watch your movements.

The following pages show the seven Basic Workout exercises for you to do. Practise these until you find them really easy.

If you do these Basic exercises correctly, you will definitely see and feel an improvement even before going on to the more advanced programmes.

Stay with the Basic Workout for one to two weeks – or as long as you need to get it right. Then continue with the Basic Workout but with the Basic Workout-Plus exercises in addition, for which you should allow an extra five minutes or more.

# BASIC WORKOUT 1

Sit or stand in front of a mirror.

Keep your back teeth together, without tension, lips slightly apart.

> *Before you begin:*
> ● *Place the pads of your middle fingers at your mouth corners on each side.*
> ● *Lightly stroke each side of your face in the direction of the arrows on the illustration, for awareness of movement.*

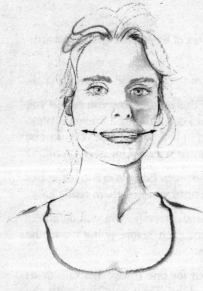

1 Grin widely, using *maximum effort* to stretch both sides of the mouth in the direction of the arrows in the illustration.
This should be one slow movement. Concentrate more on the lower lip movement – like saying '*ee*'.

2 Hold for a count of five.

3 Return slowly to the starting position.
Relax and breathe.

Do this twice only, then continue directly with Basic Workout 2.

> *Do not squint or tense your eye muscles.*

# BASIC WORKOUT 2

Sit or stand in front of a mirror.

Keep your back teeth together, without tension, lips slightly apart.

> *Lightly stroke each side of your face in the direction of the arrows on the illustration, for awareness of movement.*

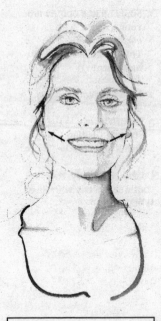

1 Smile out towards the mid-ear position, with *maximum effort.*
   This should be one slow movement.

2 Hold for a count of five.

3 Return slowly to the starting position.
   Relax and breathe.

Do this twice only, then continue directly with Basic Workout 3.

> *Do not squint or tense your eye muscles.*

# BASIC WORKOUT 3

Sit or stand in front of a mirror.

Keep your back teeth together, without tension, lips slightly apart.

> *Lightly stroke each side of your face in the*
> *direction of the arrows on the illustration,*
> *for awareness of movement.*

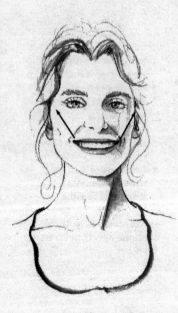

1 Smile up and out towards
   your temples, with
   *maximum effort.*
   This should be one slow
   movement.

2 Hold for a count of five.

3 Return slowly to the
   starting position.
   Relax and breathe.

Do this twice only, then
continue directly with Basic
Workout 4.

> *Do not squint or tense your*
> *eye muscles.*

# BASIC WORKOUT 4

Keep your back teeth together, without tension, lips *slightly further* apart.

> *Lightly stroke each side of your face in the direction of the arrows on the illustration, for awareness of movement.*

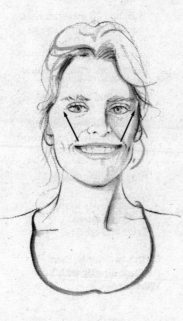

1 Raise your upper cheek muscles towards your outer eye corners, with *maximum effort*.
This should be one slow movement.

2 Hold for a count of five.

3 Return slowly to the starting position.
Relax and breathe.

Do this twice only, then continue directly with Basic Workout 5.

**Note** This upward movement is *not* a smile with the mouth corners. Try to raise the muscles towards your eye corners.

> *Do not squint or tense your eye muscles.*

# *BASIC WORKOUT 5*

Keep your back teeth together, without tension, lips relaxed.

> *Lightly stroke each side of your face in the direction of the arrows on the illustration, for awareness of movement.*

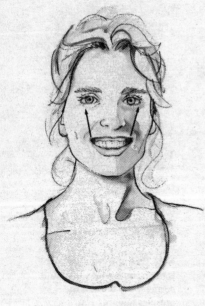

1  This time *lift* up your cheek muscles towards your eye centres, in the direction of the arrows on the illustration, with *maximum effort.*
   This should be one slow movement. You will find this easier if you move the top lip slightly in an upward direction – a semi-snarl.

2  Hold for a count of five.

3  Return slowly to the starting position.
   Relax and breathe.

Do this twice only, then continue directly with Basic Workout 6.

> *Do not squint or tense your eye muscles.*

# *BASIC WORKOUT 6*

Keep your back teeth together, without tension, lips relaxed.

> *Lightly stroke each side of your face in the direction of the arrows on the illustration, for awareness of movement.*

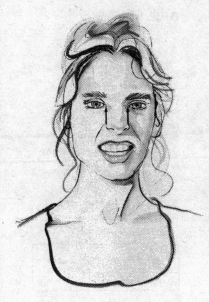

1  *Snarl* upwards with the muscles on each side of your nose, with *maximum effort*.
   This should be one slow movement.

2  Hold for a count of five.

3  Return slowly to the starting position.
   Relax and breathe.

Do this twice only, then continue directly with Basic Workout 7.

> *Do not squint or tense your eye muscles.*

# BASIC WORKOUT 7

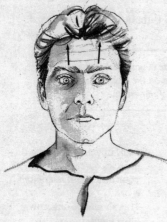

1 This time raise your eyebrows as high as you can – really stretch up with your eyes wide open.

2 Hold for a count of five.

3 Return slowly to the starting position.

Do this twice only.

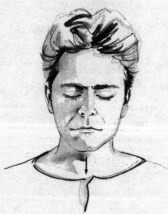

Now relax by looking downwards, with your eyes closed.
Relax your neck, your shoulders – in fact your whole being.

> *Do not squint or tense your eye muscles.*

Work through all seven Basic Workouts twice a day, so that each exercise is done four times a day in all. You will not need a mirror when you are familiar with this routine. You can do it anywhere, any time. You can do it sitting, standing, lying down – even in bed.

# THE BASIC WORKOUT-PLUS

## PROGRAMME PLANNER

Do *not* start this programme until you have thoroughly understood the Basic Workout programme and find it easy to do. When you reach that stage, continue with both the Basic Workout and the Basic Workout-Plus.

The basic Workout-Plus is very similar to the first programme except that you are working the muscles on one side of the face at a time.

So, do the next six exercises moving the muscles on the right-hand side of your face *only*.

Then repeat the exercises moving the muscles on the left-hand side of your face *only*.

Time needed: Allow ten minutes or more for the Basic and Basic Workout-Plus combined.

You may find the Basic Workout-Plus a little difficult at first, especially as one side of the face is usually weaker than the other. Keep going, though – your muscles will gradually become stronger.

Take as long as you need over these first two Workout programmes – you are not competing with anyone. However, do work out regularly – five or six days a week – to get a good result.

When you know the Basic Workout and the Basic Workout-Plus routines thoroughly and find them easy to do, go on to the Intermediate Workout programme and discontinue both the Basic routines.

# BASIC WORKOUT-PLUS 1

Sit or stand in front of a mirror.

Keep your back teeth together, without tension, lips slightly apart.

Remember – move the muscles on one side of your face *only*.

1 Move the right-hand corner of your mouth out in the direction of the arrow.
This should be one slow movement – like saying '*ee*'.

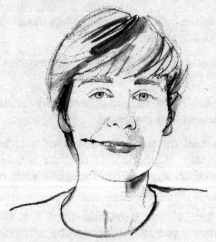

2 Hold for a count of five.

3 Return slowly to the starting position.
Relax and breathe.

Do this twice only, then continue directly with Basic Workout-Plus 2.

## *BASIC WORKOUT-PLUS 2*

Keep your back teeth together, without tension, lips slightly apart.

Remember – move the muscles on one side of your face *only*.

1 Move the right-hand corner of your
  mouth out towards the mid-ear
  position.
  This should be one slow movement.

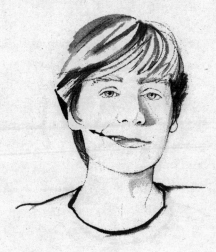

2 Hold for a count of five.

3 Return slowly to the starting position.
  Relax and breathe.

Do this twice only, then continue
directly with Basic Workout-Plus 3.

# *BASIC WORKOUT-PLUS 3*

Keep your back teeth together, without tension, lips slightly apart.

Remember – move the muscles on one side of your face *only*.

1 Smile up and out towards your right-hand temple.
This should be one slow movement.

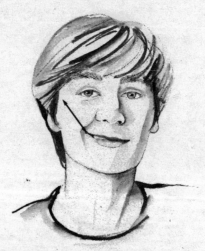

2 Hold for a count of five.

3 Return slowly to the starting position.
Relax and breathe.

Do this twice only, then continue
directly with Basic Workout-Plus 4.

## *BASIC WORKOUT-PLUS 4*

Keep your back teeth together, without tension, lips slightly
further apart.

Remember – move the muscles on one side of your face *only*.

1 Raise your upper cheek muscle towards
the outer corner of your right eye.
This should be one slow movement
from the position of the dot shown on
the illustration.

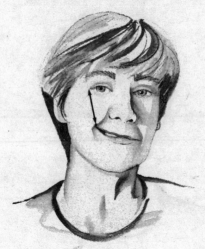

2 Hold for a count of five.

3 Return slowly to the starting position.
Relax and breathe.

Do this twice only, then continue
directly with Basic Workout-Plus 5.

## *BASIC WORKOUT-PLUS 5*

Keep your back teeth together, without tension, lips relaxed.

Remember – move the muscles on one side of your face *only*.

1 Lift your upper cheek muscle – from
   the position of the dot shown on the
   illustration – towards your right eye
   centre.
   This should be one slow movement –
   a semi-snarl.

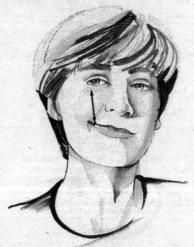

2 Hold for a count of five.

3 Return slowly to the starting position.
   Relax and breathe.

Do this twice only, then continue
directly with Basic Workout-Plus 6.

## *BASIC WORKOUT-PLUS 6*

Keep your back teeth together, without tension, lips relaxed.

Remember – move the muscles on one side of your face only.

1 Snarl using the muscle on the right-
hand side of your nose.
This should be one slow movement.

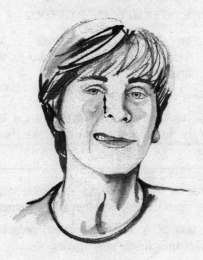

2 Hold for a count of five.

3 Return slowly to the starting position.
Relax and breathe.

Do this twice only, then repeat Basic
Workout-Plus 1–6 using the muscles on
the left-hand side of your face.

# THE INTERMEDIATE WORKOUT

## PROGRAMME PLANNER

Discontinue your Basic Workout programmes

Continue with the neck and eye warm-up exercises
as before.


### THE INTERMEDIATE WORKOUT

Time of day:   Any time (except when tired)
Time needed:   As long as it takes, once a day on five or six
              days a week

*Always sit or stand in front of a mirror.*

Start with one or two minutes of relaxation (page 8),
then go on to the Intermediate Workout exercises on the
following pages.

You will *always* need to sit or later stand (if preferred) in
front of a mirror for this Workout – you must *watch* every
movement; you must *concentrate* on every movement.

Be patient – this is a very important programme in
gaining control of the muscle movements.

When you know the Intermediate Workout exercises
thoroughly and find them easy to do, carry on with them
but do the Intermediate Workout-Plus exercises as well.

# INTERMEDIATE WORKOUT 1

This exercise will help strengthen the lower cheek muscles, mouth corners and neck muscles.

Keep your teeth and lips very slightly apart, to prevent tension.

*Before you start the exercise, place your fingertips at each of your mouth corners. Now lightly stroke each side of your face in the direction of the arrows on the illustration, for awareness of movement.*

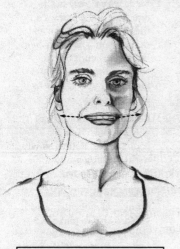

1 Move your mouth corners back in two slow movements, as follows. First move your mouth corners *half-way* back very slowly in the direction of the arrows on the illustration. Hold this position for a count of five. Then move your mouth corners back as far as possible, very slowly. Again hold for a count of five.

2 Return slowly to the *half-way* position. Hold for a count of five. Return slowly to the starting position. Relax and breathe.

3 When you find steps 1 and 2 easy, increase the number of movements until you can make five slow movements. Hold for a count of five after *each* movement. Return in the same way. Relax and breathe.

Do this twice only, then continue directly with Intermediate Workout 2.

*Concentrate more on the movement of the lower lip – rather like saying 'ee'. Work up from two to five slow movements.*

*There must be no movement or tension in the eye area.*

# INTERMEDIATE WORKOUT 2

This exercise will help strengthen the lower cheek muscles and mouth corners.

Keep your teeth and lips very slightly apart, to prevent tension.

*With your fintertips, lightly stroke each side of your face in the direction of the arrows on the illustration, for awareness of movement.*

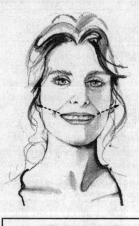

1 Smile very slowly in the direction of the arrows on the illustration, to the mid-ear position – *half-way only*. Hold for a count of five. Now continue this movement very slowly as far as you can.

2 Return slowly to the half-way position. Hold for a count of five. Return slowly to the starting position. Relax and breathe.

3 Gradually increase the number of movements until you are able to make five slow movements to the mid-ear position. Hold for a count of five after *each* movement. Return in the same way. Relax and breathe.

Do this twice only, then continue directly with Intermediate Workout 3.

*Keep relaxed during these exercises. Concentrate on at first two, slow movements without tension, then work up to five.*

*There will be slight movement in the under-eye area. However, do not squint or tense the eye muscles – they must stay completely relaxed.*

# INTERMEDIATE WORKOUT 3

The following four Workouts are to strengthen the upper cheek muscles.

By now you should find it quite easy to locate and move these muscles. Take your time – you need to gain control of the muscles at this stage.

Keep your teeth and lips slightly apart, to prevent tension.

*With your fingertips, lightly stroke each side of your face in the direction of the arrows, for awareness of movement.*

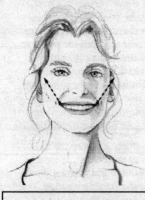

*This time we are looking for a lift in at first two slow movements, working up to five. Keep the mouth corners relaxed. Make each movement from the position of the dots towards your temples.*

*The under-eye area will crease up during this exercise. However, you must keep the eye muscles relaxed – do not squint.*

1 Raise your cheek muscles up and outwards – from the position of the dots on the illustration – very slowly *halfway* towards your temples. Hold for a count of five. Now try another lift towards your temples – again lift from the dot positions shown in the illustration. Hold for a count of five.

2 Return slowly to the half-way position. Hold for a count of five. Return slowly to the starting position. Relax and breathe.

3 Gradually increase the number of movements until you can make five slow movements in the direction of your temples. Hold for a count of five after *each* movement. Return in the same way. Relax and breathe.

Do this twice only, then continue directly with Intermediate Workout 4.

# INTERMEDIATE WORKOUT 4

These exercises strengthen the upper cheek muscles, giving an appearance of fuller, high cheek-bones.

Keep your teeth and lips slightly apart, to prevent tension.

*With your fingertips, lightly stroke each side of your face in the direction of the arrows on the illustration, for awareness of movement. Do not, however, assist the movement with your fingers.*

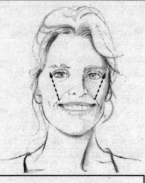

*This is very similar to Intermediate Workout 3. However, now each lift is from the dot on the illustration towards your eye corners.*

*The under-eye area will crease up during this exercise. Keep the eye muscles relaxed – do not squint. You are working the muscles from above the mouth area upwards, not the eye muscles.*

1 Raise your cheek muscles half-way towards your eye corners – from the positions of the dots on the illustration in the direction of the arrows. Hold for a count of five. Now lift the muscles again towards your eye corners. Again hold for a count of five.

2 Return slowly to the half-way position. Hold for a count of five. Return slowly to the starting position. Relax and breathe.

3 Increase the number of movements until you can make five slow lifting movements towards your eye corners. Hold for a count of five after *each* movement. Return in the same way. Relax and breathe.

Do this twice only, then continue directly with Intermediate Workout 5.

# *INTERMEDIATE WORKOUT 5*

This is again for the upper cheeks, like Intermediate Workout 4.

*With your fingertips, lightly stroke your face in the direction of the arrows on the illustration, for awareness of movement.*

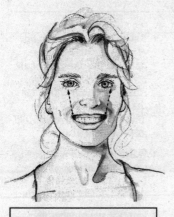

Proceed as for Intermediate Workout 4, but this time lifting towards the centre eye position, in the direction of the arrows on the illustration.

The top lip should *slightly* lift upwards, almost in a semi-snarl.

Again you may find it easier to touch the face *very lightly* with the fingertips for awareness of movement of the muscles throughout this exercise – an inch or so out from the nostrils on each side is a good position. Do *not* press or assist the movement with your fingers – it's your muscles that have to do all the work!

Do this twice only, then continue directly with Intermediate Workout 6.

*Make each movement from the position of the dot on the illustration towards your eye centres. Work up from two to five slow movements.*

*The under-eye area will crease up during this exercise. Keep the eye muscles relaxed – do not squint. You are working the muscles from above the mouth area upwards, not the eye muscles.*

# INTERMEDIATE WORKOUT 6

This is a final routine for the upper cheeks.

Keep your teeth and lips slightly apart, to prevent tension.

---

*With your fintertips, lightly stroke your face in the direction of the arrows on the illustration, for awareness of movement.*

---

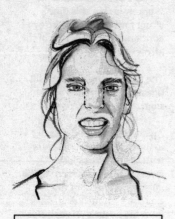

1  Raise the muscles each side of your nostrils half-way only – in the direction of the arrows on the illustration. Hold for a count of five. Lift the rest of the way in the direction of the arrows. Hold for a count of five.

2  Now return half-way. Hold for a count of five. Return to the starting position. Relax and breathe.

3  Increase the number of movements until you can make five slow lifting movements in the direction of the arrows. Hold for a count of five after *each* movement. Return in the same way.

*Lift the muscles each side of your nostrils, like a dog snarl. Work up from two to five slow movements.*

*The under-eye area will crease up during this exercise. Keep the eye muscles relaxed – do not squint. You are working the muscles from each side of the nostril up, not the eye muscles.*

Remember – these movements are like a gradual snarl. Relax and breathe.

Do this twice only, then continue directly with Intermediate Workout 7.

# INTERMEDIATE WORKOUT 7

You will have already come across this exercise in the Basic
Workout, but it should be done here too.

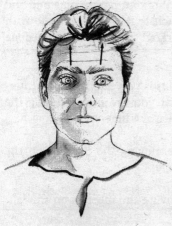

1 This time raise your
   eyebrows as high as you
   can – really stretch up with
   your eyes wide open.

2 Hold for a count of five.

3 Return slowly to the
   starting position.

Do this twice only.

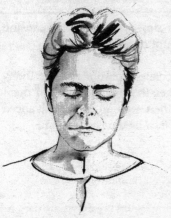

Now relax by looking
downwards, with your eyes
closed.
Relax your neck, your
shoulders – in fact your whole
being.

> *Do not squint or tense your
> eye muscles.*

# THE INTERMEDIATE WORKOUT-PLUS

## PROGRAMME PLANNER

Do *not* start this programme until you have thoroughly understood the Intermediate Workout programme and find it easy to do. When you reach that stage, continue with both the Intermediate Workout and the Intermediate Workout-Plus.

The Intermediate Workout-Plus is very similar to the Intermediate Workout, except that you are now working the muscles on one side of your face at a time.

So, do the next six exercises moving the muscles on the right-hand side of your face *only*.

Then repeat the exercises moving the muscles on the left-hand side of your face *only*.

Always move the muscles in slow, gradual steps, pausing after each movement for a count of five.

When you know the Intermediate Workout and the Intermediate Workout-Plus routines thoroughly and find them easy to do, then – and only then – go on to the Advanced Workout, which will be your *final* lifetime programme.

# *INTERMEDIATE WORKOUT-PLUS 1*

Sit or stand in front of a mirror.

Keep your teeth and lips *very slightly* apart, to prevent tension.

Remember – move the muscles on one side of your face *only*.

1 Move the right-hand corner of your mouth in five slow movements in the direction of the arrow shown on the illustration.

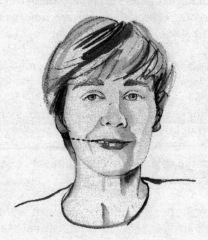

2 Hold for a count of five after *each* movement.

3 Return slowly in the same way. Relax and breathe.

Do this twice only, then continue directly with Intermediate Workout-Plus 2.

# *INTERMEDIATE WORKOUT-PLUS 2*

Keep your teeth and lips *very slightly* apart, to prevent tension.

Remember – move the muscles on one side of your face *only*.

1 Move the right-hand corner of your mouth towards the mid-ear position, in five slow movements.

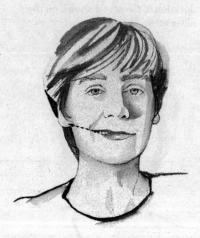

2 Hold for a count of five after *each* movement.

3 Return slowly in the same way. Relax and breathe.

Do this twice only, then continue directly with Intermediate Workout-Plus 3.

40

# INTERMEDIATE WORKOUT-PLUS 3

Keep your teeth and lips *very slightly* apart, to prevent tension.

Remember – move the muscles on one side of your face *only*.

1 Smile up and out towards your right temple in five slow movements, in the direction of the arrow.

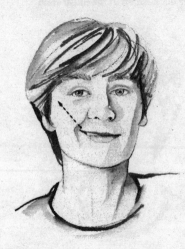

2 Hold for a count of five after *each* movement.

3 Return slowly in the same way. Relax and breathe.

Do this twice only, then continue directly with Intermediate Workout-Plus 4.

## *INTERMEDIATE WORKOUT-PLUS 4*

Keep your teeth and lips *very slightly* apart, to prevent tension.

Remember – move the muscles on one side of your face only.

1 Raise your upper cheek muscle towards the outer corner of your right eye, in five slow movements, all from the dot position in the illustration.

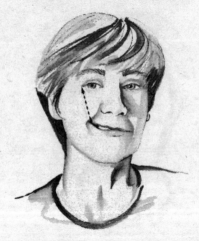

2 Hold for a count of five after *each* movement.

3 Return slowly in the same way. Relax and breathe.

Do this twice only, then continue directly with Intermediate Workout-Plus 5.

# INTERMEDIATE WORKOUT-PLUS 5

Keep your back teeth together without tension, lips relaxed.

Remember – move the muscles on one side of your face *only*.

1 Lift your upper cheek muscle towards the centre of your right eye, in five slow movements, all from the dot position in the illustration.

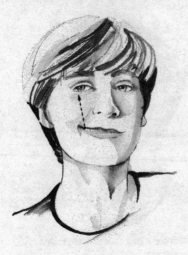

2 Hold for a count of five after *each* movement.

3 Return slowly in the same way. Relax and breathe.

Do this twice only, then continue directly with Intermediate Workout-Plus 6.

# INTERMEDIATE WORKOUT-PLUS 6

Keep your back teeth together without tension, lips relaxed.

Remember – move the muscles on one side of your face *only*.

1 Snarl up with the muscle on the right side of your nose, in five slow movements in the direction of the arrow.

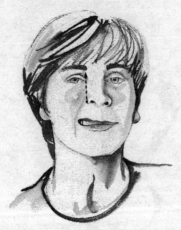

2 Hold for a count of five after *each* movement.

3 Return slowly in the same way. Relax and breathe.

Do this twice only, then repeat Intermediate Workout-Plus 1–6 using the muscles on the left-hand side of your face.

44

# THE ADVANCED WORKOUT

Discontinue all previous Workouts

This is your lifetime programme.

In this group of exercises you will be working
the muscles against a resistance. As you
know, lack of exercise makes the muscle
tissue become thin and wasted. Working the
facial muscles against a resistance will help to
bring back the elasticity and tone to the muscle
tissue, making it plump and strong again.

You will need to put aside time each day really
to study and practise this final stage. You may
find that working the muscles against a
resistance is difficult at first – nothing seems to
move. But be patient – you will begin to find it
easier from day to day, and then quite soon it
will become simple.

Do, however, find time quietly on your own
really to relax and concentrate on getting
it right.

Take your time over the Advanced Workouts –
choose a few of the ones that you need most
(they are all listed at the front of the book) and
practise those, adding others as you become
competent.

Don't take on too much at first, or you may find
that you haven't time to do any of it properly.

# PROGRAMME PLANNER

Do *not* start this programme until you are completely
competent in carrying out the Intermediate Workouts and
Intermediate Workout-Plus. When you reach that stage,
give up those Workouts and continue with the Advanced
Workouts only.

If you start the Advanced Workouts too soon, you will find
it impossible to move your muscles against the now
necessary resistance.

Continue with your neck and eye warm-up exercises
as before.

### THE ADVANCED WORKOUT

Time of day:  Any time (except when tired)
Time needed:  While learning – as long as it takes, once a
day on five days a week
When experienced – about ten minutes a
day, three days a week

You will now need a pair of cotton cosmetic gloves (or two
pieces of thin cotton fabric or soft tissues) and also some
Vaseline to lubricate the under-eye area.

The gloves or fabric are essential, to prevent your fingers
slipping when holding the muscles against resistance.

Always exercise with a clean skin – no make-up or creams
– but use Vaseline to lubricate the under-eye area *only*. Do
not use eye creams or gels for this purpose.

Apply the Vaseline with the pads of your middle fingers, starting at your temples and lightly smoothing downwards then under the eyes towards the bridge of your nose.

The Advanced Workout programme must be followed with total relaxed concentration and *always in front of a mirror*. When experienced you may sit or stand, but always work out in front of a mirror.

Start with one or two minutes of relaxation (page 8), then carefully carry out the instructions on the following pages for the Advanced Workouts that you have selected.

Do each Workout three times.

**Remember:**

● Always choose a time when you are not in a hurry.

● Always exercise in front of a mirror.

● Always watch and concentrate on every movement.

● Always exercise with a clean skin – no make-up or creams.

● Always use Vaseline to lubricate the under-eye area only.

# TO BUILD AND STRENGTHEN THE UPPER CHEEK MUSCLES

This exercise and stages 2 and 3, which follow, are to strengthen the upper cheek muscles. When fit and strong, these muscles give the face an enormous lift.

Nose-to-mouth lines and folds will gradually lessen, and the underlying tissue will strengthen, giving a fuller, more youthful appearance.

You will need to sit in front of a mirror with your elbows resting on a table.

You should be looking *straight ahead* into the mirror.

You may have to rest your elbows on a raised support, so as not to bend forward too much.

It is important to be relaxed and comfortable throughout this Workout.

Don't rush – one step at a time, in the long run, is the quickest way to achieve your goal.

# TO BUILD AND STRENGTHEN THE UPPER CHEEK MUSCLES – STAGE 1

Wearing gloves, sit in front of a mirror, with your elbows resting on a table.

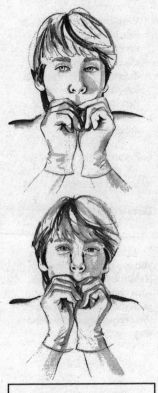

1 Place the flats of your thumbs in each side of your mouth, between your teeth and your cheeks.

2 Hold on outside with the side of your curved index fingers, knuckles facing each other.

3 Curve your thumbs slightly forward. Keep your hands steady and hold them down slightly.

4 Now lift the muscles on each side of your nose in three small movements against the resistance of your grip. Pause after *each* movement for a count of five.

5 Return in the same way. Relax and breathe.

Do this three times.

*Never allow your hand/ finger resistance to move up with the muscle lift – you are working the muscles against the hold.*

When you have understood and perfected these movements, proceed to Stage 2.

# TO BUILD AND STRENGTHEN THE UPPER CHEEK MUSCLES – STAGE 2

Follow Stage 1, steps 1–4, then proceed as follows:

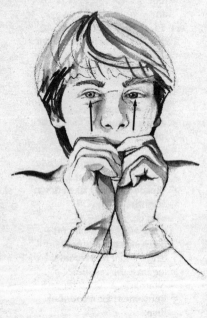

5 With the muscles on each side of your nose lifted, now lift the rest of your cheek muscles in the direction of the arrows in five slow movements. Remember to pause for a count of five after *each* movement.

6 Return in the same way.

Relax and breathe.

Do this three times.

To sum up, at this stage you are making a total of eight movements upwards, with counts of five after each movement. You are then returning in the same way.

*You must keep very relaxed throughout the Workout – tension will make it difficult to move the muscles.*

# TO BUILD AND STRENGTHEN THE UPPER CHEEK MUSCLES – STAGE 3

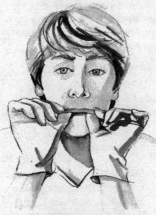

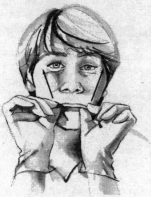

1 Place the flats of your thumbs in each side of your mouth, between your teeth and your cheeks.

2 Hold on outside with your curved index fingers – this time with the palms facing towards the mirror, as shown in the illustration.

3 Curve your thumbs slightly forward. Keep your hands steady and hold them down slightly.

4 Now lift your upper cheek muscles half-way, in the direction of the arrows. Hold for a count of five, then lift the muscles the rest of the way and again hold for a count of five.

5 Return in the same way. Relax and breathe.

Do this three times.

---

*When you start this Workout, lift in only* two *movements, gradually increasing the number to* five *as you are able to.*

Increase the number of movements until you can make five slow movements in each direction, each from the previous holding position, with a pause for a count of five after *each* movement.

# TO STRENGTHEN THE UPPER EYELIDS

Lack of exercise can cause the eyelids to droop considerably, making the eyes look smaller and the lids go into folds with drooping corners. Working the eyelid muscles can give a much more youthful and alert appearance.

Look *straight ahead* into a mirror throughout this exercise.

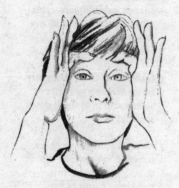

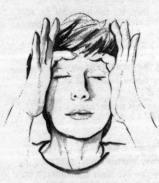

1 Curve your index fingers under your eyebrows. Hold each side of your head with your thumbs.

2 Push up your eyebrows and hold them firmly against the bone. It is important to keep this firm hold throughout.

3 Close your eyelids very slowly, feeling a good downward pull from brow to lashes.

4 Now squeeze your eyelids together really tightly. Hold for a count of five.

5 Release the squeeze slowly for a count of five.

6 Open your eyelids. Relax and breathe.

Do this three times.

> *It is important to keep a firm hold throughout.*

# TO STRENGTHEN THE UNDER-EYE MUSCLES – STAGE 1

Strengthening the under-eye muscles will help to eliminate lines, bags and puffiness in the under-eye area.

You will need Vaseline on your under-eye area, applied as described in the Programme Planner.

For this exercise you may find it easier to *stand* in front of a mirror – one that's attached to the wall and extends slightly higher than the top of your head.

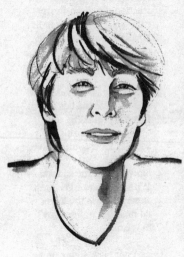

Now lean towards the mirror, with your hands resting on a table or wash-basin to steady you.

Watch your eyes in the mirror. Then very slowly lift the lower lids upwards in tiny movements.

This is not easy, but it can be done. At first try just two movements up and two movements down. Gradually increase to five movements each way.

Do this three times.

As you lift the lower lid you will notice that the muscle movement goes upwards towards the bridge of the nose. This is correct.

Practise these up and down movements until you can make the five movements up and five down while remaining relaxed.

*After the fifth movement your lids should be almost shut. All movements are from the lower lids only. When you have achieved this, continue with the next stage.*

# TO STRENGTHEN THE UNDER-EYE MUSCLES – STAGE 2

With Vaseline on your under-eye area, stand in front of a mirror.

Rest your hands on a table or wash-basin to steady yourself.

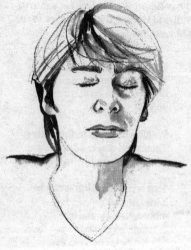

1 Lean forward slightly and look into the mirror.

2 Raise your eyebrows fractionally, then slowly raise your lower lids in five small movements to half-close your eyes – as though squinting into the sun.

3 Now close your eyes gently and squeeze the lids tightly together, relaxing your eyebrows. Hold this tight squeeze for a count of five.

4 Slowly relax the squeeze. *With your eyes still closed,* slowly release the lower lid muscles, in five slow movements.

Open your eyes. Relax and breathe.

Do this three times.

*Be careful not to scowl.*

*Remember to lift your lower lids until almost shut before closing your eyes.*

# TO STRENGTHEN THE LIPS AND THE SURROUNDING MUSCLES

The three exercises that follow will work-out the muscles surrounding the mouth. The benefits are enormous.

As we age, the lips and surrounding areas can become very thin and wizened. The resulting lined and sunken effect can add years to one's appearance.

These exercises will help to rebuild the muscles around the mouth, giving a fuller, more youthful appearance.

# TO STRENGTHEN THE LIPS AND THE SURROUNDING MUSCLES

Sit or stand. Look into a mirror. Feel relaxed.

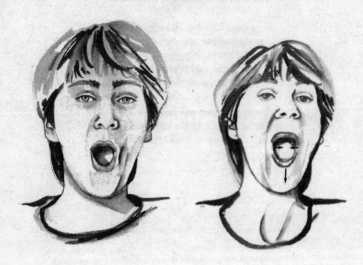

1 Open your mouth slightly as if to yawn (about a 1-inch gap).

2 Now lower your *jaw only* in eight *slow* movements, at the same time gradually moving the corners of your mouth inwards.
After the eighth movement your mouth must form an *oval* (not a round) shape. Your lips and the surrounding areas should feel very taut at this stage, with your jaw dropped down as far as possible.

## TO STRENGTHEN THE LIPS AND THE SURROUNDING MUSCLES

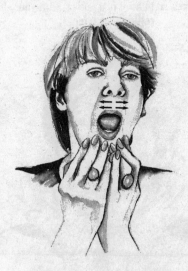

3  In this position, place your fingers on your chin area as shown in the illustration and gently hold it down.

4  Now stretch your top lip, in the direction of the arrows, in five small movements, keeping your mouth an oval shape.
Hold for a count of five.

5  Return in five small movements, then relax your upper lip, remove your fingerhold on your chin and relax.

Do this three times.

# TO ERASE LINES ON THE UPPER LIP

Wearing gloves, sit in front of a mirror, with your elbows resting on a table.

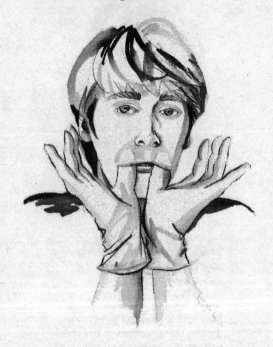

1 Place your thumbs under your top lip, your thumb-nails resting against your gums.

---

*The space between your thumbs must remain the same throughout.*

---

## TO ERASE LINES ON THE UPPER LIP

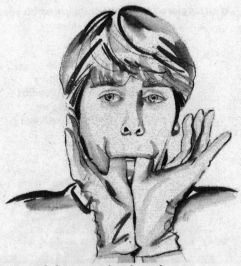

2 Now, feeling very relaxed, gently move your upper lip muscles towards your thumbs in eight small movements.

3 With your upper lip muscles very firmly pressed against your thumbs, hold for a count of five.

4 Keeping your thumbs in the same position, release your muscles in eight slow movements.

Relax and breathe.

Do this three times.

# *TO STRENGTHEN THE LOWER LIP*

Wearing gloves, sit in front of a mirror, with your elbows resting on a table.

1 With your teeth about 1 inch apart, hook the first joint of your index fingers behind your lower lip, with your finger-nails resting slightly forward from your lower teeth and gums.

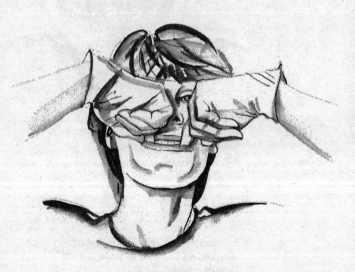

> *Finger resistance must remain rigid throughout.*

## *TO STRENGTHEN THE LOWER LIP*

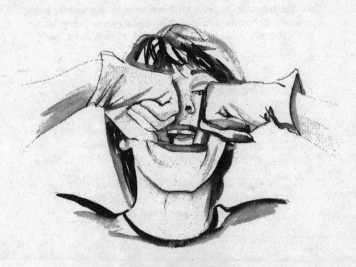

2  Pull your lower lip and chin muscles
   in against the finger resistance, in
   eight small movements.

3  With your muscles very firmly
   contracted against your fingers, hold
   for a count of five.

4  Keeping your fingers in the same
   position, release your muscles in eight
   slow movements.

Relax and breathe.

Do this three times.

# TO STRENGTHEN THE CHIN MUSCLES

As we age, the muscles of the chin can weaken and shrink, giving a general pinched, sunken look. This again can be prevented by strengthening these muscles, leading to a fuller, more toned appearance.

Look into a mirror – feel relaxed.

Keep your teeth together, lips relaxed.

1 Move the centre of your lower lip and your chin muscles downwards in one very small movement.

2 Place your fingertips *lightly* on your chin area as shown in the illustration. Your fingertips should just meet.

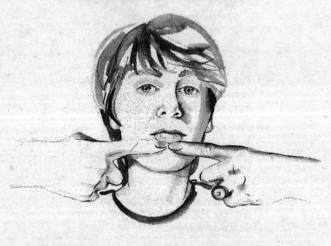

Do not smile out with your mouth corners.

## TO STRENGTHEN THE CHIN MUSCLES

> *All movements are from the centre of your
> lower lip and chin.*

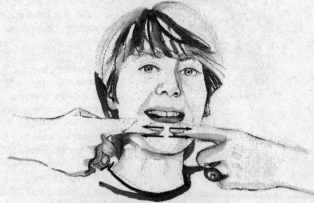

3 Now move your lower lip and chin
muscles outwards in the direction of
the arrows in eight slow very small
movements.

4 Hold for a count of five.

5 Return in eight very slow movements.

Relax and breathe.

Do this three times.

In this exercise the fingers are used simply to feel the stretch of
the chin muscles outwards.
The fingertips will part with each muscle movement, leaving an
eventual gap of about $\frac{1}{2}$ inch. At Stage 5 they will gradually meet
up again.

# TO EXERCISE THE MUSCLES OF THE NECK AND JAW LINE

Leave this exercise out if you have any jaw problems.

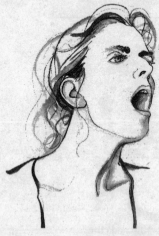

1 Sit or stand with a straight spine. Tilt your head up and back slightly. Now jut out your chin.

2 In this position, keeping your head still, open your mouth wide by lowering your jaw. Now grin widely.

3 Bring your back teeth together gently. Now – still grinning – lower and raise your jaw ten times.

Relax and breathe.

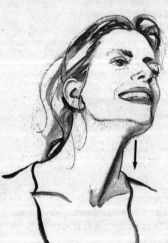

> **DOS**
> *Keep the wide grin position throughout. Concentrate on the lifting of the jaw.*

> **DON'TS**
> *Do not gnash your teeth together. There should be no tension in your forehead. There should be no tension in your eye area.*

This exercise should be performed *only once* daily.

# TO FIRM THE MUSCLES UNDER THE CHIN AND HELP ELIMINATE A DOUBLE CHIN

*Don't hold your fist too firmly against your chin – it is there as a gentle resistance.*

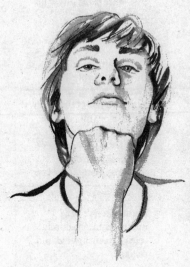

Sit in front of a mirror.

1 With your back teeth together, without tension, jut your chin forward and *very slightly* upwards.

2 Rest your elbows on a table. Place your clenched fist under your chin. Put bottom lip forward and raise up over top lip.

3 Now press the *tip* of your tongue against the roof of mouth (about $1\frac{1}{2}$ inches back from your front teeth). The *tip* of your tongue should do all the work, gradually increasing the pressure slowly during a count of five. Wait for a few seconds.

4 Slowly release the pressure during a count of five.

Relax and breathe.

Do this three times.

*Don't squint – keep your eyes relaxed.*

# TO HELP ELIMINATE JOWLS AND IMPROVE THE JAW LINE AND NECK

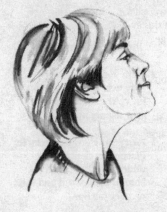

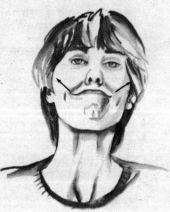

Stand or sit in front of a mirror.

1  Tilt your head up and jut your chin forward.

2  Slide your upper lip down behind your lower teeth. Gently grip your upper lip with your teeth.
   (If this is difficult for you, just place your lower lip over your top lip.)

3  With a stretched feeling in the front of your neck, slowly smile up and out in the direction of the arrows in five slow movements.

4  Hold for a slow count of five, gently stroking upwards along your jaw line.

5  Return in five slow movements. Gradually release your liphold and relax.

Breathe.

Do this three times.

> *You should feel a good pull around your jaw line and throat.*

# TO SHAPE AND SLIM THE LOWER CHEEKS

This exercise will help make the lower part of your face slimmer. If your need the reverse, leave out this exercise and turn to the next page.

1 Smile upwards vigorously.

2 Keeping your upper cheeks as high as you can, bring your lips forward and pout (not pucker) them.

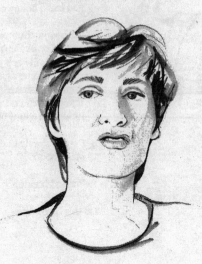

3 Now make rapid kissing noises ten times, keeping the lower cheeks sucked in.

Do this three times.

# TO FILL OUT HOLLOWS IN THE LOWER CHEEKS

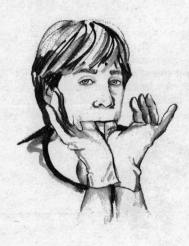

Sit or stand in front of a mirror.

1 Place your thumbs inside your mouth, between your back teeth and your cheeks.

2 Place the pads of your thumbs outwards against your cheeks – anywhere you feel a hollow.

3 With your thumbs firmly pushed out against your cheeks, pull back your cheek muscles against your thumb resistance in eight small movements. Hold for a count of five.

4 Return slowly in eight small movements.

Relax and breathe.

Do this three times.

## *TO PREVENT AND HELP ELIMINATE SCOWL LINES*

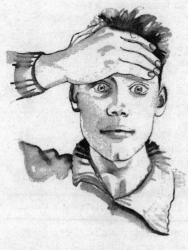

Sit or stand in front of a mirror.
Look straight ahead.

1 With your eyes open, gradually widen them in five slow movements. Do not move your eyebrows. (It may be helpful to hold your eyebrows still by placing the palm of your hand on your forehead.)

2 Pause for a count of five. Then return in five slow movements.

3 Close your eyes and look down.
Totally relax.
Breathe.

Do this three times.

*Do not blink throughout.*
*Do not raise your eyebrows.*

You can repeat this exercise several times a day
(if you wish).

This exercise will help to prevent not only scowl lines but also crow's-feet at the outer corner of your eyes. It is mainly squinting that causes these problems. Make it a habit to keep your eyes wide open but relaxed.
Do not stare.

# TO ELIMINATE
# EXPRESSION LINES

Smear a small amount of Vaseline over
the lines. Then with the pads of your
middle fingers, press firmly over the
lines, rocking your fingers from side to
side for a count of ten or more.

You can do this several times a day, if
you wish.

Lines will gradually fade if you observe
the following rules:

1 Stop squinting – squinting causes
  crow's-feet and lines under the eyes.
  Keep your eyes wide open and relaxed
  – not staring – and practise the
  exercise for scowl lines (page 69).

2 When you smile, don't screw up your
  eyes. Smile by moving your mouth
  corners towards your ears – this is a
  natural smile. Do not smile up
  towards the eye corners.

3 Don't knit your brows together.
  (See the exercise for scowl lines on
  page 69.)

4 Don't raise your eyebrows, except
  when exercising. Practise palming
  (page 154) – stay totally relaxed in
  your brow and eye areas.

**Note** You will find other remedies for
facial lines in the chapter on massage.

# TO ELIMINATE LINES ON THE BRIDGE OF THE NOSE

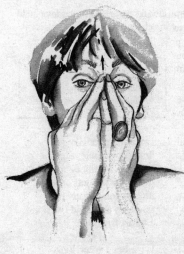

1 Place your middle fingers *each side* of the bridge of your nose. Hold firmly and down slightly.

2 Now place your third fingers on the *top* of the bridge of your nose, just below any lines or bumps.

3 Gradually move the muscle between your fingerhold in the direction of the arrows, in five tiny slow movements.

4 Hold for a count of five. Then slowly return in five movements.

Relax and breathe.

Do this three times.

---

*The finger resistance must be held gently but firmly throughout.*

*Feel relaxed – do not scowl.*

---

# TO ELIMINATE HORIZONTAL LINES ON THE FOREHEAD

Sit in front of a mirror, with your elbows resting on a table or held against your chest.

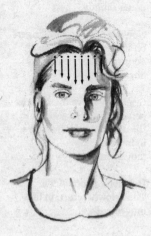

> *All the movements must come from the top of the forehead downwards.*

1 Place the pads of your fingertips along your hairline, on the points marked with dots on the illustration. Gently push upwards and hold the skin against the bone.

2 With head erect, look straight ahead. Now try to bring your brow down in five movements against the resistance of your hold, gradually closing your eyes.

3 Hold this downward pull for a count of three, then slowly release. Relax and breathe.

Do this three times.

> *Do not scowl.*
> *Do not push your head into your hands – this will cause tension at the back of your neck.*

# MAKE-UP AND HAIR

This is not a beauty book in the usual sense, but make-up is fun and, used properly, is a great confidence-booster for many. The problem is that books, magazines and television programmes often give conflicting advice – the result very often being a shelf full of cosmetics that we never use.

It can be useful to take a personal lesson at a make-up school or salon, testing out the various products for your skin tones. However, always wait before buying any of the products chosen for you, in case you find that you don't really like that particular look after all when you get home. You will be given a list of the preparations used – buy the ones you want at a later time.

The three models in the photographs on the following pages all look good before as well as after make-up. Whichever look you prefer, it is marvellous to have this choice. They were made up by Vanessa Haines, who believes in enhancing rather than disguising features. The make-up was applied surprisingly sparsely and yet gives a very sophisticated look.

Please read through this section – it may be helpful. As the weeks go by, you will certainly notice a difference when applying make-up on a firmer, fitter face – it's so much easier!

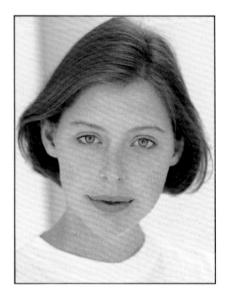

Before beginning your make-up, make sure
you start with a clean face. Take a good look at
yourself and decide what you need in the way of
make-up and what look you are aiming to
achieve.

Use a light moisturizer, but *do not* apply it on
the under-eye area. Instead, use a *tiny* smear of
vaseline – gently remove any surplus with a
tissue.

# CONCEALER

Lighten the dark areas of the face with the concealer, taking care to hide high-colour blemishes and spots. Use concealer sparingly, as it contains much more pigment than ordinary foundation. If you have naturally good skin, concealer, blusher and powder may be all you need.

Pat rather than rub concealer into the skin, remembering to blend it in well with your foundation. Always choose a colour that will blend in well with your skin tone.

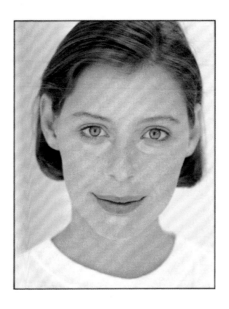

# FOUNDATION

Find the correct type and colour of foundation for your
skin. The make-up counters of many of the better
department stores will advise on the right
colour for you.

You can apply foundation with a sponge or with your
fingers, the latter being more hygienic. If you do use
a sponge, make sure it is kept clean – dirty sponges
lead to dirty skin and, in some cases, skin infections.

Apply foundation, a little at a time – you can always
add more, but taking some away is more difficult.
Your foundation should never feel like a mask. You
may not even need to apply it all over the face,
so really study yourself first.

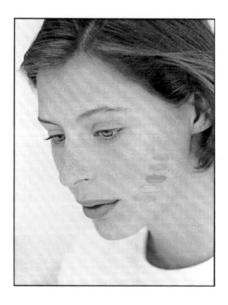

## BLUSHER AND POWDER

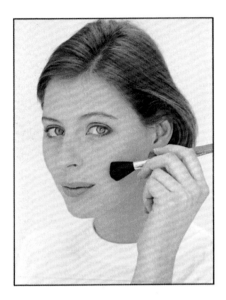

Use loose powder on a brush to set your foundation.

Blusher should give the face a natural glow. Gone are
the days of streaks of pink or red up the sides of your
face – rather than making you look slimmer in the
face, these age and date you. Blush your cheeks to
look as if you had caught the sun a little, making you
look healthy.

The colour of your cheeks should complement the
colour of your lips, so make sure you have a couple of
different shades of blusher to hand – a pink to match
the red and pink lipsticks, and a peach tone to match
the browns and corals. When you have brushed your
cheeks with blusher, blend well with loose powder.

# *EYES*

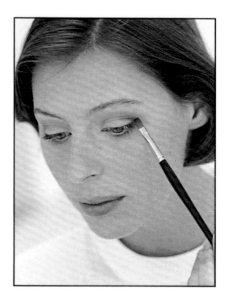

It is a good idea to experiment with lots of different colours of eye make-up, to find those that enhance the colour of your eyes. Many women get stuck in a rut, with blue eye-shadow or black kohl around the eyes. Try doing without these – the change can be miraculous.

Eye-shadow should enhance your eyes, not overpower them. Avoid bright colours – always use muted shades. Experiment, but remember that the colour of your eyes should be more prominent than your eye-shadow.

# *LIPS*

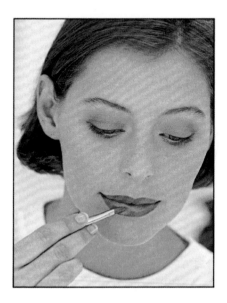

Make sure that lips are well looked after from the start, especially in extremes of heat and cold. Lip-liners can be a good idea, but see that they are blended in to the lip colour – harsh lines can look very overpowering. Lip-liners can help to contain the lipstick and so prevent the colour bleeding on to the skin.

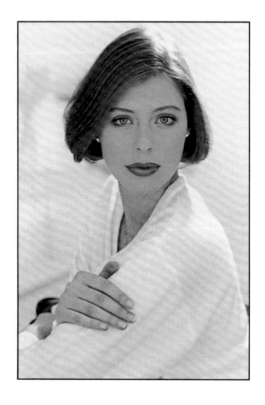

If you want a line under your eyelashes, make sure
you smudge well with an earthy tone of eye-liner
(pencil) or powder eye-shadow on a good-quality
brush – hard lines detract from the eye. You don't
have to take the line all the way under the lashes –
take it half-way from the outer corner, being careful
to blend.

*Amanda looks marvellous with or without make-up and with straight or curled hair – as you will see.*

After applying a light foundation, set it with loose powder. Take a large brush, dip it into the powder, then tap the brush on the back of your hand, bristle side down, to break up the particles, before lightly dusting the powder all over your face.

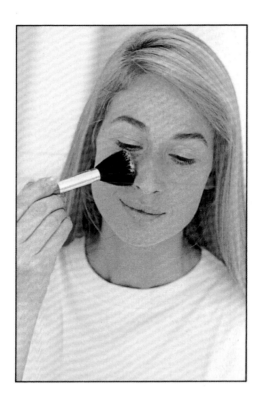

Brush your eyebrows upwards, as this makes a good frame for the eyes. If you need to darken your eyebrows, try to darken just the hairs rather than the skin, to avoid having a painted-doll look. You can use a soft eyebrow pencil or a dark powder on a firm brush.

If you are blonde or a redhead, colour your eyebrows only a little, otherwise the effect can look too harsh.

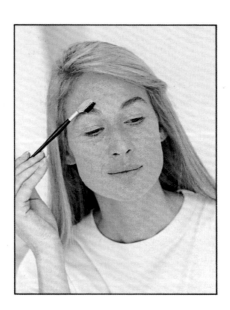

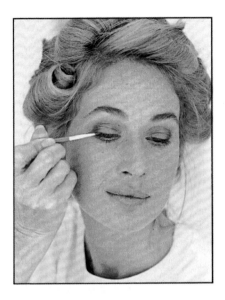

If you have deep-set or small eyes, use a darker shade
on the outer corners of the eyes then sweep colour a
shade lighter across the lids. This widens the eyes.
This technique will look good on almost anyone.
Merge the lashes into the lids with a very thin drawn
or painted eye-line.
In the socket, brush in a light line in a mustard or
peach shade. (You could use your blusher for this.)
Experiment with all colours, as I said before, but I
feel that the more natural shades enhance the eyes
more than brighter colours.

If your eyes are very large or protrude, make sure
that the darkest area is at the centre of the lid and
fade the colour away from this in each direction. Try
to avoid shiny or glittery eye-shadows – they
emphasize problem areas and can cause eye
irritations if wrongly applied.

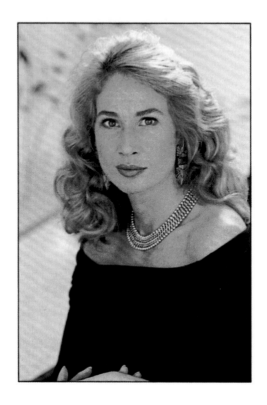

*With this very simple, light make-up Amanda goes on to ring the changes with a new hairstyle.*

*Amanda has the sort of hair that goes into any style. With a few rollers, she achieves this completely different look.*

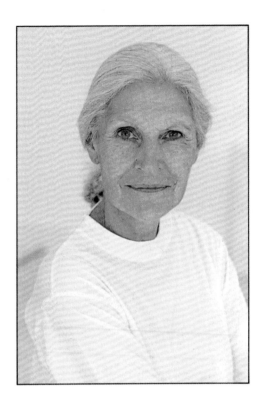

*Here, we have Pam, who enjoys wearing carefully
applied make-up.*

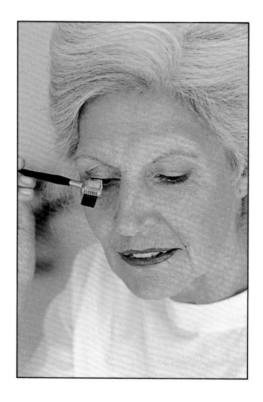

Mascara should not be applied like a coating of glue!
Make sure you wipe excess mascara from the brush
before you start, so that you get a clean coating on
your lashes. You can then comb through the lashes
to get rid of any excess mascara.

You can achieve a good effect by applying mascara to
the top lashes only. Applying it to the bottom lashes
as well can make them look spidery.

Blotting the lips can be a good idea, to get a more
subtle look. Split three-ply tissue for this, so that you
don't take too much colour off. Always apply a second
coat of lipstick for more staying power. Again,
blot lightly.

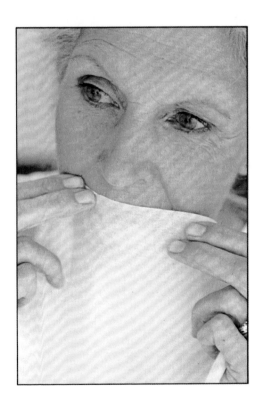

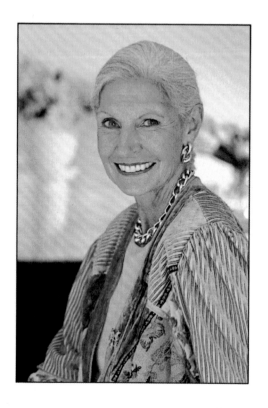

Lipstick is very important here – it enhances Pam's
marvellous smile.
Pam's eye make-up is muted eye-shadow – grey in
this case – just on the lids. No highlighter has been
used, as it can be very ageing.

# DIET

## FOOD INTOLERANCE AND ALLERGIES

In using the word 'diet', we are not necessarily concerned with a restricted food intake for slimming purposes but with our overall food consumption. There is no doubt that what we eat and drink plays a great part in how well we feel.

If you feel well, energetic and cheerful then you are obviously on the right track. If the reverse is true, however, then it is a good idea to check your diet.

Some people may experience depression as a result of intolerance to a particular food – not necessarily one of the 'bad' foods but just as often something that is considered quite harmless.

I know two people who recently found the cause of periodic bouts of depression that they had been suffering for years. In one case these had been caused by eating grapefruit; in the other by eating peaches. Once these foods were left out of the diet, the people concerned began to live their lives free of the previous terrible spates of despondency.

Many rheumatic complaints can be made worse by an intolerance to certain foods. Tomatoes are suspect for many people, for example. Gelatine may also have the same effect – even such small amounts as the gelatine capsules for vitamins and minerals. Obviously, these substances do not affect everyone, but it is worth checking on every intake of food and drink, however small, to save further suffering.

Of course this should not stop you consulting your doctor if you do not feel well, but some of us, at the same time, could do far more to help ourselves than we may realize.

If you have periodic ups and downs in health, it is useful to write down *everything*, however minute, that you eat and drink over a period of weeks. You will soon notice if there is any relationship between what you eat and how you feel.

Stomach complaints can be caused through eating dairy foods or wheat produce. If you have stomach problems, try eating products made with oatmeal, rice or rye instead of wheat – see if this makes any difference.

Coffee, tea and colas are often drunk automatically without any check of the consequences. These substances seem to do very little harm to many of us. To others, however, they are destructive drugs. I always suggest that, before asking your doctor for tranquillizers or the like, you should try restricting your intake of these drinks. You might be amazed at the effect such a reduction could have on your well-being, without resorting to pills. I am not saying you should cut out these substances altogether, but if you think you may be suffering unwelcome side-effects you should not consider this state of affairs to be natural. Check them out for yourself.

If particular foods or drinks seem to be causing problems, cut whatever they are out of your diet for a while, then experiment to find out at what level you can tolerate them. You may not have to give them up altogether.

There are clinics that specialize in food tolerance tests and investigating allergic reactions to foods. However, if you have the patience, you can determine any food allergies yourself – it takes very little time each day.

## LOSING WEIGHT

Anyone who has a real weight problem has probably tried many of the endless diets on the market by now, perhaps successfully for a time, only to regain all the lost weight very quickly later. Crash diets inevitably end this way.

Unfortunately, when dieting – which for some people means all the time – food is constantly in your thoughts.

How many calories have you consumed? How many calories have you left? What are you eating at your next meal? What are you eating tomorrow or next week? So, just when you should be forgetting about food and getting on with your life, the reverse is happening.

It is not easy to solve the problem of rapid weight gains and losses, but think about this: if you lost just 1 lb ($\frac{1}{2}$ kg) a week, in one year you would be 52 lb (26 kg) lighter. A small minority have that amount or more to lose; most probably have 20 lb (10 kg) or less excess weight. By losing 1 lb ($\frac{1}{2}$ kg) a week, you could lose 20 lb (10 kg) in 20 weeks – with a greater likelihood of keeping the weight off.

These slow weight-loss regimes are tedious, though – most of us want to see quick results, even if in a few months we are back to square one. However, I really believe that the only way to keep weight off is through slow, steady weight loss, which means *not* giving up all the foods that make mealtimes enjoyable, as this usually leads to a craving for these foods. Try eating meals you would normally eat, but cut down considerably on the fat and sugar content. You need not even make endless lists, which again cause more concentration on food.

There are five types of nutrient that your body needs (in addition to water and dietary fibre): proteins, carbohydrates, fats, vitamins and minerals. These last two will be discussed in the next section.

Proteins are essential for building and repairing body tissue. Meat, poultry, fish, eggs, milk, cheese, dried beans, lentils, nuts and seeds all contain proteins.

Protein is essential, but your daily requirement is surprisingly small. If you eat more protein than your body requires, it is converted into body fat. On average, 4 oz (115 g) a day is adequate.

Carbohydrates are divided into two basic types: complex and simple. Simple carbohydrates provide quickly released energy, the main source being sugar as in sweets, chocolate desserts, cakes, biscuits, soft drinks, etc.

Complex carbohydrates provide long-term energy: sources include whole-grain cereals, bread, pasta, rice, potatoes, vegetables and fruit.

Complex carbohydrates should account for at least 55 per cent of your food intake. Yes – potatoes, bread, vegetables, etc. are all allowed, but not the foods containing simple carbohydrates, like cakes and biscuits.

Fats may be of vegetable or animal origin. Animal fats are found in such things as butter, lard, whole milk, beef, lamb, and pork. Vegetable fats include oils such as olive oil, sunflower oil, corn oil, etc. and also margarines.

The fats in food are of three different types: saturated, mono-unsaturated and polyunsaturated. ('Saturated' means that the fat contains as much of the element hydrogen as it can, 'mono-unsaturated' means that it contains less, and 'polyunsaturated' means that it contains less still.) There has been much conflicting advice about which fats and oils are good for you and which are not. Heart disease and cancer are still on the increase despite the reduction in the use of saturated (mainly animal) fats, and some experts blame the over-use of polyunsaturated oils for the disturbing statistics.

Polyunsaturates are health-giving if used wisely but should be selected with care if to be used for heating or cooking, as some of them break down and start to foam or smoke at lower temperatures than others. Blended vegetable oil and corn, grape seed, groundnut, rape seed, safflower and sunflower oils are the most suitable for shallow and deep frying (if you must) and for brushing on to food before grilling or roasting. Extra virgin first pressing olive oil is more suitable for use in salad-dressings than in cooking, although other oils such as grape seed, sunflower and safflower can also be used for salad-dressings if you prefer a less pronounced taste. Store all oils in a cool dark place. For spreading, use low-fat, high-in-polyunsaturates spreads, rather than butter.

Animal fats are best avoided – try to keep to vegetable oils (but *not* coconut oil or palm oil). However, a low fat intake is essential while trying to lose weight. (Some fat intake is necessary, though, so that the body can absorb the fat-soluble vitamins, such as vitamins A, D and E, which we shall discuss later.) Reduce your salt intake too, especially if you are inclined to retain water or if your ankles sometimes swell. If you do resort to a diet book, choose one that recommends a low fat intake.

Try cutting out all fried foods, and cut down on solid fats like butter and margarine.

Cutting down on biscuits, cakes, sweets and chocolates will automatically reduce your sugar intake. Just lessening your taste for these particular items can in itself cause you to lose weight steadily over the months.

Drink plenty of water each day – six glassfuls (3 pints or 1.7 litres) is a good amount.

One thing you will need to do in order really to succeed is to exercise. Any form of exercise will do, as long as you work out for twenty minutes continuously. Walking, swim- 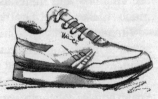 ming, keep-fit routines or an exercise bike are all excellent. Twenty minutes twice a day is even better. The Basic Body Movements to Fitness chapter in this book will give you some ideas.

Exercise will make you feel fitter and it also helps to strengthen your will to succeed. If you do slip up on occasions, though, don't make that an excuse to try again 'some time'. Don't forget that you are not dieting as such; you are simply cutting down considerably on the foods that are not really good for you anyway.

Remember, if you really want to lose weight, you will do so eventually, no matter how often you have tried and failed in the past. On the other hand, if you are not the lean type and have no wish to be – if you are really happy at the weight you are and it does not impair your health – then you should stay that way whatever others say or think to the contrary. Following fashion is pointless if it is not what you want. Being too thin can be just as harmful to your health as being overweight, even though it's fashionable.

At the end of the day, to be well, fit and healthy should be your main concern.

## *VITAMINS AND MINERALS*

As well as proteins, carbohydrates and fats, discussed in the previous section, the other important types of nutrient are vitamins and minerals, though these are required in much smaller quantities than the others.

Vitamins are involved in regulating body processes, and so all of them contribute to healthy growth and development.

Minerals are also necessary for normal bodily processes. For example, calcium contributes to the physical structure of bones and teeth and plays a part in muscle contraction and blood clotting; iron is a constituent of the compound that carries oxygen in the blood to the cells where it is used in the release of energy from nutrients such as carbohydrates.

A balanced diet that includes a variety of different types of food is likely to contain adequate amounts of all the vitamins and minerals that the body requires. However, it is possible for deficiencies of particular vitamins to occur; pregnant or nursing women have an increased need for vitamins, for example, and strict vegetarians and others on restricted diets may not receive adequate amounts of all vitamins. Mineral deficiencies may also occur – iron-deficiency anaemia being perhaps the most common. In such cases a vitamin or mineral supplement may be useful, and we will look at the possible need for particular vitamins and minerals below.

The number of vitamin and mineral supplements on the market is vast and can be very confusing. Mineral supplements vary enormously, and not all multivitamins contain the same ingredients. Many contain cheap ingredients which will be poorly absorbed and which can also cause serious disorders. They may be packed with unnecessary additives, fillers, binders and colourings and may be covered with detrimental sugar coatings. Cheap, badly formulated supplements are not effective and are therefore a waste of money.

So, when using supplements, follow two very general rules.

First, never supplement individual nutrients on their own. For example, if you need vitamin B6, don't take it without the support of a good B-complex vitamin supplement. If zinc is necessary, for example, take it as part of a top-quality multivitamin/mineral complex. Indiscriminate self-medication of isolated nutrients can do more harm than good and may, in the long term, actually cause deficiencies of other nutrients in the body. If you cannot find a multivitamin/mineral supplement which contains exactly what you need, seek advice from a pharmacist or homoeopath – do *not* take individual vitamins or minerals in addition to a multivitamin/mineral supplement.

Second, buy good-quality products from reputable suppliers. Don't be fooled by exaggerated advertising or biased media reporting. Nothing is a cure-all, and no single substance has the power to make a significant difference to symptoms without the support of other complementary nutrients, a sensible and moderate diet, and a gentle but regular exercise programme:

- Include plenty of nature's greatest convenience foods in your diet: fresh green and root vegetables, salads, fresh fruits, peas, beans and lentils. Avoid the skins of fruit and vegetables unless you know they are organic, and always wash them thoroughly before use to remove as much as possible of any chemical spray.

- Keep dairy foods to a minimum. Seek out organic and free-range products.

- Keep fried foods to an absolute minimum, and avoid rich cakes, biscuits and junk food.

- Diets containing large amounts of protein should be viewed with caution. Avoid red meat if you can and stick to fresh fish and free-range poultry.

- An adequate fluid intake is vital, and this means drinking plenty of fresh (preferably filtered) water, but avoiding excessive amounts of tea, coffee and colas. Try to drink at least 3 pints (1.7 litres) of fluid each day between meals.

- And of course, take regular exercise.

Together, these simple actions will help to encourage the removal of toxic deposits in the body, improve elimination of harmful waste and increase the shedding of old cells and the growth of new ones.

All the nutrients which feed the body work together in a way which is greater than the total of their individual effects, but extra supplies of certain individual nutrients can make an enormous difference to skin quality, as we shall see.

### VITAMIN A

Vitamin A is an essential skin nutrient and is found in the diet in two basic forms: retinol, which is vitamin A itself and is found only in foods of animal origin, and beta-carotene, which occurs in some foods of plant origin and is converted to retinol during digestion.

Beta-carotene is an important anti-ageing nutrient. Good sources of beta-carotene include orange and yellow vegetables and fruits such as carrots and apricots, cantaloup melons, parsley, watercress and all green, leafy vegetables.

In ideal conditions the body will convert beta-carotene to vitamin A in the small intestine and liver. However, there is growing concern among nutritionists that a large percentage of the population may not be able to effect this conversion efficiently enough to absorb adequate quantities of vital vitamin A. For example, diabetics and those suffering from digestive disorders and malabsorption problems have problems absorbing vitamin A in this way.

Retinol – the vitamin A available from animal food sources such as liver, fish liver oils, eggs and dairy produce – can be toxic if used incorrectly, so it would be wise to take professional advice on supplementation where a deficiency is suspected or additional amounts are thought to be required.

For general use, the recommended daily intake of retinol is 7500 I.U. (international units). Larger amounts of beta-carotene are regarded as safe – up to 20,000 I.U. daily.

Both retinol and beta-carotene are widely available from food sources, and yet vitamin A remains one of the most commonly deficient vitamins in the British diet. If you have one or more of the following symptoms, you might benefit from taking a vitamin-A supplement: frequent and recurring skin infections; acne; dry or scaly skin; throat infections or mouth ulcers; thrush or cystitis; dandruff; night-blindness; sore, itchy, burning or inflamed eyelids; dry hair.

## THE B VITAMINS

There are eight vitamins in the vitamin-B complex: thiamine (B1), riboflavin (B2), niacin (B3), folic acid, biotin (vitamin H), pantothenic acid (B5), pyroxidine (B6) and cobalamin

(B12). These vitamins are essential in many ways, not least in the production of energy, the rebuilding of tissue and the nourishing of the nervous system. Particular foods are rich in particular B vitamins, but liver is a good source for all of them, eggs (especially the yolks) and whole-grain cereals for many, and vegetables and pulses for some.

Deficiency symptoms are myriad but can include the following: premenstrual syndrome; irregular, heavy or painful periods; menopausal imbalances; cracks, sores or splits around the nose and the mouth; tingling or burning sensations in the limbs; lack of energy, anaemia and pale – generally poor – skin condition. The B vitamins are usually found to be lacking where there are skin problems.

If necessary, take a good-quality B-complex supplement which contains 50 mg of each B vitamin – preferably 'enzyme-activated', to facilitate absorption.

## VITAMIN C

Vitamin C is necessary for the body's immune response to infections and in wound-healing, and is also essential for maintaining the strength of blood capillaries and for the formation of collagen – often referred to as the glue that holds the skin together. Collagen degeneration can be a sign of vitamin-C deficiency, and when the elasticity of collagen collapses, skin can age very quickly. Other signs of a diet lacking in vitamin C are frequent colds and infections, bleeding gums, cystitis, constipation and broken veins.

Vitamin C is found in most fresh fruit and vegetables. Good sources are citrus fruits, tomatoes, potatoes and green, leafy vegetables; strawberries and cantaloup melons contain large amounts. Significant amounts of vitamin C can be lost during boiling and if food is kept hot for a long time before serving. Some is also lost in excessive washing and cutting of foodstuffs.

If necessary, take a good-quality vitamin-C complex – containing bioflavonoids – at 2 grams (2000 mg) daily.

## VITAMIN D

Vitamin D helps in the absorption of calcium from the intestinal tract and so is essential for strong bones and teeth.

Good sources of vitamin D include oily fish (such as sardines, herring, tuna and salmon), liver, milk and dairy products and egg yolks. It is also formed by the action of the ultra-violet rays in sunlight on chemicals naturally present in the skin.

The small amounts of vitamin D required daily are usually adequately provided by a balanced diet and normal exposure to sunlight, but supplements are sometimes necessary for those with inadequate exposure to sunlight, for strict vegetarians and for the elderly. Long-term deficiency can lead to softening of the bones, with associated backache, muscle weakness, bone pain and fractures.

Except for initial treatment of deficiency symptoms under medical supervision, the maximum daily dose of vitamin D should not exceed 400 international units – prolonged excessive use can lead to a variety of adverse effects, including weakness, unusual thirst, depression and abnormal calcium deposits within the body.

## VITAMIN E

The vitamin to reduce scarring following accident or surgery, vitamin E is known to prolong cell life, improve skin quality and hasten wound-healing. Clinical trials have proved its effectiveness in the treatment of heart disease, hormonal imbalances and hypertension. If you bruise easily or have very dry skin, vitamin E can make a real difference.

Vegetable oils are good sources of vitamin E, as are green, leafy vegetables, whole-grain cereals and wheatgerm.

If you use a lot of polyunsaturated vegetable oils, though, you could benefit from taking extra vitamin E.

Do obtain professional guidance on supplementing vitamin E, however – it is a fat-soluble nutrient, stored by the body, and can be dangerous if prescribed incorrectly or in the wrong quantity. If you decide to use it, keep to below 400 international units daily. With best-quality vitamin-E supplements – which are structured to be more biologically active in the body – as little as 100 I.U. will be sufficient.

## ESSENTIAL FATTY ACIDS

Sometimes known as the vitamin-F complex, essential fatty acids (EFAs) are just that – essential. They cannot be produced by the body and so they must be provided in the diet.

Essential fatty acids have many vital functions within the system. They are active in the structure of cell membranes; they increase oxygen uptake and they are an important component in energy production. The balance of hormones within the body is adversely affected by a deficiency or malfunction of fatty acids, as is muscle tone. Clinical research has proved their great value in the treatment of existing skin conditions and in maintaining healthy skin.

Dietary sources of EFAs are limited. Fish oil and linseed oil can provide derivatives of one important kind of fatty acid from the 'omega-3' family. Evening primrose oil is a well-known member of the family known as 'omega-6 triglycerides', providing a substance called gamma linoleic acid (GLA).

If you need essential fatty acid supplements, it is important to look for good-quality products. Safe and effective ones will not be cheap, so, as a very general rule, buy the most expensive you can afford. If you choose evening primrose oil, the recommended dose is between 150 mg to

250 mg daily or four to six capsules containing around 8 per cent GLA per capsule. There are pure GLA complexes available which give 16 per cent, so you take less – but avoid those derived from borage oil, which are not well absorbed by the body. There are a few supplements avail-able which offer a mixture of omega-3 and omega-6 triglyc-erides in the same capsule.

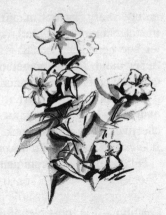

It is best to avoid essential fatty acids sold in liquid form. Many have been subjected to oxygen contamination during the bottling process and will therefore have no beneficial effect on the body. Even those that are produced under stringent conditions will have a very short shelf-life.

## PROBIOTICS

Together with the kidneys, liver, lungs, lymphatic system and bowels, the skin is one of the body's major means of waste elimination. When one of these systems is sluggish, the othes will try to make up for it. This is one of the reasons why the skin will erupt so readily if, for example, constipation is a problem or there is overloading of the lymph system – the organs which drain tissue fluid back into the bloodstream and fight infection.

The digestive tract contains bacteria which have many beneficial effects on the healthy activity of the gut and are particularly important in the maintenance of healthy skin. Apart from assisting in the removal of toxic build-ups in the body, their natural antibiotic activity helps to boost immu-nity, inhibit the growth of undesirable bacteria and promote the production of vitamin A from beta-carotene. Unfortunately, many factors in our modern life-style – including the over-use of antibiotics – make it more and more difficult for the beneficial, health-giving bacteria to maintain the upper hand. Nature sometimes needs a little help, and this is where probiotic supplements can be of enormous benefit.

There are many different kinds of probiotic supplement available. Most have similar names, but some are more effective than others. Look out for those which contain *Bifidus* and *Lactobacillus acidophilus*.

Follow the pack recommendations for dosage.

## CALCIUM

Calcium is the most plentiful mineral in the body, making up over 90 per cent of the hard material of bones and teeth. It is essential for the formation and maintenance of strong bones and healthy teeth and also for the contraction of muscles, for the transmission of nerve impulses and for blood clotting.

The main sources of calcium in the diet are milk and dairy products; sardines; dark green, leafy vegetables; dried beans and nuts. In hard-water areas, calcium may also be obtained by drinking tap water.

Unless sufficient dairy products are consumed, the diet may not contain enough calcium and so the body is forced to obtain the calcium it needs from the skeleton. This is not evident in the short term, but in the long term this can lead to fragile bones (osteoporosis), backache, muscle weakness, bone pain and fractures. Severe deficiency leading to low calcium levels in the blood can cause cramp-like spasms in the hands, feet and face. Women are particularly susceptible to calcium deficiency, as pregnancy and breast-feeding require large amounts of this mineral.

The recommended daily dietary allowance of calcium for adults is 800 mg (or 1200 mg during pregnancy or breast-feeding). A pint of milk contains about 600 mg. If sufficient is not obtained from the diet, supplements will be necessary. Calcium is usually supplemented alongside vitamin D, which helps its absorption from the intestine.

Although osteoporosis has been linked to calcium deficiency in some cases, this may not be helped by supplements in all women.

## IRON

Iron is involved in the formation of red blood cells and forms part of the compounds which carry oxygen in the blood to the cells where it is used in the release of energy from nutrients (such as carbohydrates) and those which store oxygen in the blood for use during exercise.

The best dietary source of iron is liver. Other good sources include meat (especially offal); eggs; chicken; fish; green, leafy vegetables; dried fruit; whole-grain or enriched cereals, breads and pasta; nuts and dried pulses. Iron from meat, eggs, chicken and fish is absorbed better than that from vegetable sources.

Most diets provide adequate supplies of iron, but heavy menstrual periods or chronic blood loss through diseases such as peptic ulcers may result in a deficiency, causing anaemia, with symptoms such as fatigue, pallor, shortness of breath and palpitations. Recommended daily dietary allowances of iron are 10–18 mg for adults.

## IODINE

Iodine is necessary for the thyroid gland to produce the hormones that control the body's energy production, promote growth and help burn excess fat. Seafood is the best source, but most people's iodine intake comes from bread and dairy produce.

Iodine deficiency may result in a goitre – an enlargement of the thyroid gland which often results in a flabby swelling of the neck – or a shortage of thyroid hormone, which may cause tiredness, physical and mental slowness, weight gain, facial puffiness and constipation.

The recommended daily dietary allowance for adults is 150 micrograms and most diets contain adequate amounts, so supplementation is seldom necessary, although iodine is a constituent of several multivitamin/mineral supplements.

### POTASSIUM

Potassium is essential for storage of carbohydrates in the body and in breaking them down for energy.

Green, leafy vegetables, oranges, potatoes and bananas are the best sources of potassium in the diet, although lean meat and pulses are also rich in it. However, many methods of food processing result in lower potassium levels than in fresh food.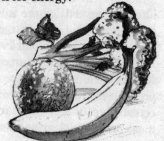

There is no official recommended dietary allowance of potassium, but 2–6 grams has been suggested as a daily intake. Most diets contain adequate amounts, however, and supplementation is seldom necessary, although potassium is available in a number of multivitamin/mineral supplements. Marginal deficiency may be caused by consumption of large amounts of coffee, alcohol or salty foods, though. Over-use of laxatives may also lead to deficiency – early symptoms may include muscle weakness, fatigue, dizziness and mental confusion.

### SELENIUM

This mineral is needed only in tiny amounts but is, nevertheless, essential. Its functions include the maintenance of elasticity in the skin (in association with vitamin E), so slowing down the ageing process. It also promotes stamina by improving the supply of oxygen to the heart muscles and it contributes to protection against high blood pressure and abnormal blood clotting which might lead to a stroke or heart attack. Surveys have shown that selenium is frequently deficient in patients with cancer and heart disease.

Good dietary sources of selenium include fish and whole-grain cereals. If supplementation is necessary, 100 micrograms daily should be sufficient.

## ZINC

Zinc is essential for the manufacture of proteins and the genetic material of cells in the body and is involved in the body's use of carbohydrates. It is also necessary for the healing of burns and wounds.

Protein-rich foods such as lean meat and seafoods are the best dietary sources of zinc, although whole-grain cereals and dried pulses are also good sources. Zinc from animal sources is better absorbed than that from plants, though.

Some authorities believe zinc deficiency to be epidemic. Symptoms include excessively dry or excessively oily skin, acne, slow wound-healing, white marks on the fingernails, persistent infections, poor hair quality and infertility. Diabetics have a higher requirement for zinc, and pregnant and lactating women should supplement zinc – it is one of the few nutrients lacking in breast milk.

Food additives can adversely affect the absorption of zinc, as can too much of the wrong kind of cereals. It is probably wiser to choose whole-grain rye, rice, oats, buckwheat and millet rather than wheat bran and wheat-based cereals.

Where necessary, supplementation of zinc is usually recommended at between 15 mg and 25 mg daily, as an ingredient of a multivitamin/mineral pill.

# THE SKIN AND WHY IT AGES

There are many reasons why the skin ages, some of which explain why it is often the more exposed areas – the face, neck and hands – which suffer the worst.

Causes of aged skin include the following:

- Too much sun. Skin depends on its moisture content, and too much sun can lead to a dried-out skin and cause permanent damage. Results – cracks in the skin tissue and irreparable deep lines.

- Harsh winds and cold, which lead to weather-beaten skin.

- Certain cleansers in the form of detergents and soaps.

- Exposure to pollution in the atmosphere.

- A poor diet – this is a main factor.

- Too much alcohol or caffeine.

- Cigarette smoking.

- Poor sleep patterns.

- Lack of exercise.

As you see, exercise is not the only factor in keeping the skin healthy, but it does play a major part. Exercise, in my experience, *can* reverse the ageing process. The results of working out the body are well known, so it stands to reason that the facial contours can benefit from exercise too.

The skin has three main layers, each attached to its neighbour. The *hypodermis* is the lowest layer of the skin. It is mainly composed of muscle and fatty tissue, and it differs considerably in thickness from one person to another. The hypodermis is usually thicker in women than in men, giving the female form its more rounded shape.

Serious illness or starvation can cause the fatty tissue of the hypodermis almost to disappear, leaving only the top two layers of skin. An overweight person, through having an excess of this fatty tissue, sometimes has a more youthful countenance and a smoother skin.

The *dermis* is immediately above the hypodermis and consists of a fibrous mass known as 'connective tissue'. This tissue is composed of two types of material: *collagen*, which is grouped together in twig-like bundles, and *elastin*, which makes up only about 2 per cent of the total but gives the skin its pliancy.

The dermis is of paramount importance. It contains the nerve endings of the skin, which give us the sense of touch, pain, heat and cold; blood vessels; lymph vessels; the hair follicles; the sweat glands and sebaceous glands, which secrete a substance called sebum which is mainly responsible for the skin's natural oils.

Exercise is important here – bringing improved blood flow, circulation of lymph and fluids to and from the cells and elimination of toxic wastes. These improvements brought about through exercise have an enormous effect on the skin, flesh and muscle and are in themselves anti-ageing.

The outer skin layer – the *epidermis* – is supported by the dermis, which acts rather like a cushion.

The epidermis consists of many layers of cells. New plump cells, known as 'basal' cells, are constantly being produced in the innermost part of the epidermis and work their way up towards the surface of the skin. Here they lose their moisture, become flatter and are shed as dead skin cells. These surface cells are tough and scaly, being rich in a substance called 'keratin' which is also the main constituent of nails and hair.

The skin on the face is attached to the facial muscles by the delicate connective tissue. It is important to keep this connection intact, so pushing and pulling of the facial skin should be avoided. Massage of the face other than through the surface stroking routines described later in the book is not recommended. During your Workout programmes, the facial skin and muscles are moved as one, so these programmes are harmless and can only strengthen and build the link between the skin and muscles. (Incidentally, massage of the body is excellent, as the skin and muscles of the body are not connected together like those of the face.)

## SKIN CARE

There are many creams on the market which help to improve the texture of the skin. They can protect the skin from some of the pollution, wind, heat and cold to which it is exposed and, to a certain extent, from the sun's rays. There are also products to help relieve surface dryness and to make the skin feel less taut, and therefore more comfortable, but I have yet to discover a miracle cream that can give you everlasting youth!

When using any skin preparation, don't just look for a softer skin. This, in my opinion, is no good at all. You should be aiming for a firmer, smoother skin.

Some products with a high oil content are so softening that, even after one application, you can see a definite droop in your features after only a few hours. Other creams cause puffiness, which can't be good. Observe any reactions to preparations applied to your face, and leave alone any preparations that seem to produce adverse effects. Aim to keep your face firm and fit.

The most important thing is to keep the skin clean. It is vital to cleanse the skin – both night and morning – particularly at night, in order to remove grime, dirt and pollution, excess oil, perspiration and stale make-up. Without proper cleansing, pores become blocked, causing blackheads and dull-looking skin.

In the morning, cleanse and/or rinse the skin to remove oil and perspiration and any accumulated dead skin cells.

Many people use a soap-and-water routine throughout their lives, and their skins can be as clear and fresh-looking as those of people who use a more complicated regime. However, some soaps can be harsh, stripping the skin of its protective acid layer and so making it feel dry and taut. If you do prefer to use soap and water, though, there are many pH-balanced soaps or foaming lotions on the market which are worth experimenting with.

It is very important always to rinse the skin thoroughly with warm water after washing, to remove every trace of any suds – thirty splashes with clear water is not too many.

No matter what cleanser you use, *never* leave the skin wet or moist afterwards: it is very important to dry the skin thoroughly. Spraying water on the face is very popular, but you must still dry the face afterwards.

If your skin feels dry after washing then you should use a creamy cleanser or a lightweight milky cleanser instead. Tissue off after application, and repeat until thoroughly clean.

If you wear make-up, you will definitely need to use a creamy or milky cleanser, even if you wash with soap and water afterwards. You would need to wash your face too many times with soap and water alone to remove all traces of make-up, and this would be too drying for any skin type.

Toners are often considered a must after using a cleanser, but I find that they tend to dry out the skin. There are cleansers on the market which are water-soluble, and I much prefer this kind – after cleansing you then need only rinse your skin thoroughly with warm water.

If you must use a toner, find one that is very mild, whatever your skin type. Follow with a thorough rinsing with cold water.

Finishing with cold water splashes produces excellent results for me, but this is not a good idea if tiny red veins are a problem.

Never use iced water on your face and neck, and certainly not ice cubes. I know that ice cubes are a popular beauty treatment, but in my experience they are extremely harmful to the skin tissue in the long run.

At night, when you have cleansed your skin by whatever method you prefer, your skin should feel smooth and fresh. If it is taut or dry – or both – then you are definitely using the wrong product, which is why so many people have to use a nightcream on a regular basis. You should sleep with a clean skin, free from creams and potions. Try using a cream at night only on the occasions when your skin really needs it.

Vaseline is an excellent lubricant and moisturizer for the skin. Apply it to a very clean skin over the entire face, leave for ten minutes and then tissue off. Splash your face with cold water and pat it dry thoroughly. Vaseline is also a marvellous under-eye lubricant. I have yet to find a cream or eye gel to surpass this, and I would never use anything else.

With all the pollution and grime in the atmosphere, it makes sense to wear some protection for the skin during the day. Make-up can be effective for this purpose, as well as being fun to wear for those who enjoy it. I love wearing make-up and find it very protective to the skin surface, but there are many other protective products you can use if you feel that make-up is not for you.

It is always difficult to advise on the use of skin preparations – it really is a question of trial and error. There are many good products on the market and when you have found the ones that give excellent results for you then you should keep to them.

As I have explained, the top layer of the skin consists of dead skin cells. These are mainly removed by cleansing, but sometimes they can stick to the surface, causing the skin to look dull. The pores can also become blocked, and dryness can become a problem.

These dead cells can be gently removed by using one of the many exfoliant preparations on the market. There are creams, gels and pastes which contain tiny granules to get rid of these cells. Using one of these once a week should be sufficient.

Another method, which I prefer, is simply to rub a soft towel over the skin's surface, making brisk circular movements over the cheeks, sides of nostrils, forehead and brows. Keep this up for about one minute every morning at first, *before you use anything on your face*. After five days, you need do this only once or twice a week. Follow this procedure with your usual morning routine. Your face should feel really vibrant using this method. Try it and see.

# BASIC BODY MOVEMENTS TO FITNESS

You may already have your own special routine for working out each day, but, in case you haven't, here are some simple exercises to get you started, so that you can progress to a fitter life-style from here on.

Try to get used to doing some body exercises every day – it soon becomes a habit, and an excellent one at that. Of all the anti-ageing formulas on the market, keeping fit and in shape surely must come at the top of any list.

Fortunately, there is no age barrier – you can start a 'getting into shape' programme at any time of life. At the extreme, look at the marathon runners who have started training in their sixties and have managed to complete the twenty-six miles. I am not advising you to go as far as this, though – I prefer walking, myself – but it does prove that age need not be a handicap.

Take a look at the following pages and choose the exercises you feel are for you – or, better still, try them all and then work out your own fitness programme.

## *A WAKING-UP EXERCISE*

On waking, lie on your back and stretch
in every direction.

Stretch your legs and feet. Wiggle your
toes. Curl your toes under and squeeze
tightly. Now stretch them apart.
Stretch out with your arms and start
yawning. Yes – yawn as much as you
want, stretching all the time.

Breathe in and out.

*As you breathe in*, feel the breath as if
starting in your toes and working up
through your body to the top of
your head.

*Now breathe out*, reversing the breath
from the top of your head through your
body to your toes.

Do this breathing several times.

Now stretch again and get up.

# TO STRETCH THE WHOLE BODY

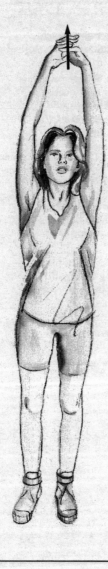

1 Stand erect, arms at your sides, feet slightly apart.

2 Raise your arms straight above your head. Clasp your hands together.

3 Now stretch your arms up as high as you can in eight movements.
You will feel the stretch in your arms, chest, abdomen, hips and thighs.
Relax slowly.

Do this stretch three times in all.

*This is an excellent exercise to do if you have been sitting for any length of time. Remain sitting to do it if you prefer.*

# TO FIRM THE MUSCLES AT THE BACK OF THE UPPER ARMS

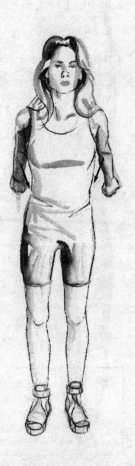

1 Stand with your legs slightly apart, your arms at your sides.

2 Clench your hands loosely, with your fingers facing the back wall.

3 Now straighten your arms backwards as far as possible for a count of five.

Do this three times.

# TO WORK OUT THE HANDS, ARMS AND SHOULDERS

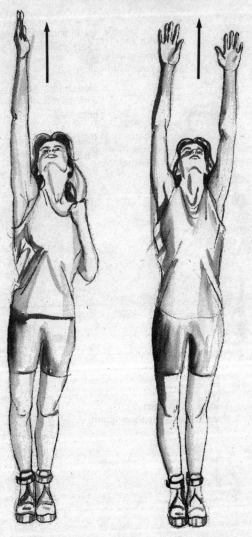

## *TO WORK OUT THE HANDS, ARMS AND SHOULDERS*

1 Stand erect with your feet together.
   With your upper arms against your
   body, clench your fists at shoulder
   level.

2 Stretch up with your right arm,
   spreading your fingers as much as
   possible. Look up at your hand and
   stretch for a count of five.

3 Return to the starting position,
   clenching your fist.

4 Repeat with your left arm.

5 Now stretch up with both arms,
   spreading your fingers apart. Look up
   at the ceiling and stretch for a count
   of five.
   Return with clenched fists to the
   starting position.

Do this three times.
Breathe regularly throughout.

## *ARM-STRETCHING EXERCISES*

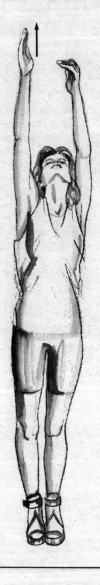

1 Stand erect, with your feet together.

2 With your arms straight above your head, stretch with your right arm as high as possible, then stretch with your left arm.

3 Now stretch up with both arms. *Really* stretch.

Do this three times. Breathe and relax.

# TO EXPAND AND STRENGTHEN THE CHEST MUSCLES

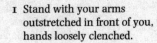

1 Stand with your arms outstretched in front of you, hands loosely clenched.

2 Swing your arms apart and back as far as possible – your right arm raised to shoulder height, your left arm lower at hip level – hands open, fingers spread.

3 Do this three times. Then do the same three times with the left arm raised and the right arm lowered.

These movements should be fairly rapid, with a good stretch each time. Do this five times.

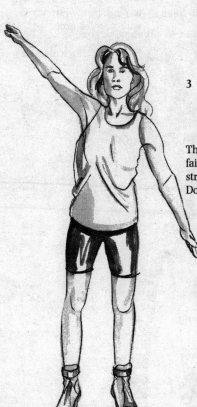

# TO STRENGTHEN THE ARM AND CHEST MUSCLES

1 Stand erect, with your feet slightly apart, your arms straight out to the sides at shoulder level, palms facing upwards.

2 Make small circles with your arms, increasing to large circles.

3 Now return to small circles.

Do this three times, in a continuous flow.

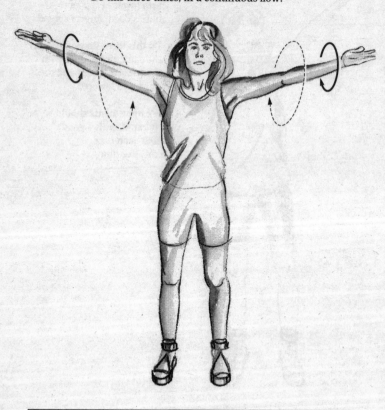

# AN EXERCISE FOR THE ARMS, SHOULDERS AND SIDES

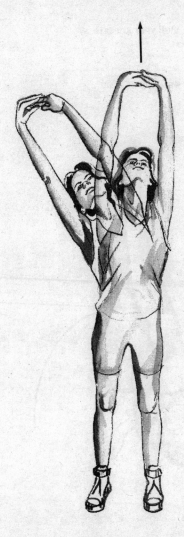

1 Stand with your feet apart. Clasp your hands above your head, palms upwards, and stretch towards the ceiling.

2 From the waist, bend to the right, keeping your arms stretched.

3 Return to the centre and, from the waist, bend to the left, arms stretched.

Do this three times.
Relax and breathe.

# TO STRENGTHEN THE STOMACH MUSCLES

1 Lie on your back. Pull your knees in towards your chest.

2 Thrust your legs straight out at an upward angle.

3 Slowly lower your legs to the floor.

Do this five times.

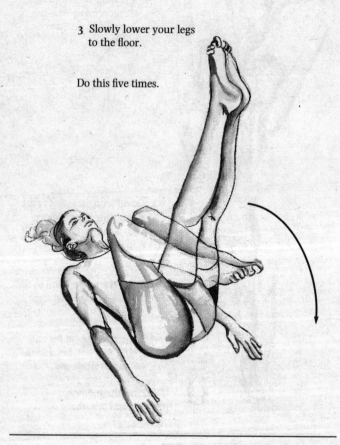

# AN EXERCISE FOR THE WAIST AND SIDE MUSCLES

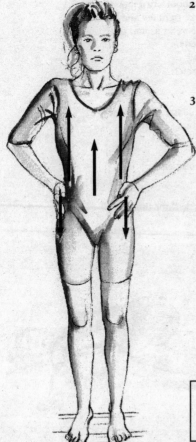

1 Stand with your feet almost together, hands resting on your hip-bones.

2 Breathe in. Press down on your hips, at the same time stretching your waist and side muscles up towards your shoulders. Really stretch these muscles.

3 Relax and repeat twice more.

*This exercise is excellent if you've been sitting for a while and feel cramped.*

# TO STRETCH THE HIPS AND WAIST

1 Lie on your back with your arms out to the sides. Bend your elbows at right angles, palms facing upwards.

2 Keeping your shoulders flat on the floor, bend your right leg and lower it to the floor (or as far as you can) across your body.
Straight left leg.
Feel a good stretch.

3 Return to the centre, then to the starting position.

4 Repeat with your left leg.

Do this whole cycle three times in all.

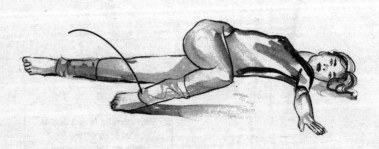

# TO FIRM THE INNER THIGHS

This exercise is easy – and it works!

1 Lie on your back, legs straight up, feet
   pointing towards the ceiling.

2 Spread your legs out to the sides as
   far as possible.

3 Return to the starting position.

These movements must be done rapidly
– as often as you wish.

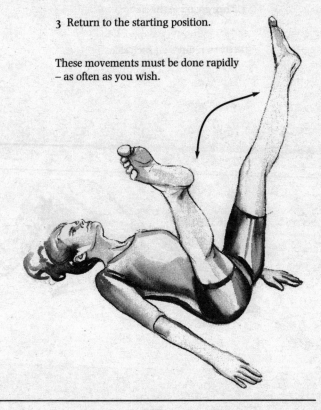

# TO REDUCE THE HIPS AND THIGHS

1 Lie on your back, knees bent, arms out to the sides.

2 Keeping your knees together, swing them over to the left, until your left leg touches the floor. Make sure both shoulders stay flat on the floor.

3 Then swing to the right.

Do this ten times on each side.

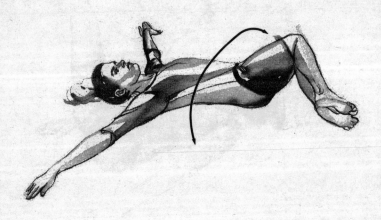

## FOR A FIRMER BOTTOM

1 Sit on the floor, legs straight in front of you, arms folded across your chest.

2 In this position, 'walk' forward on your buttocks – ten steps forward, then ten steps back, or as far as space allows.

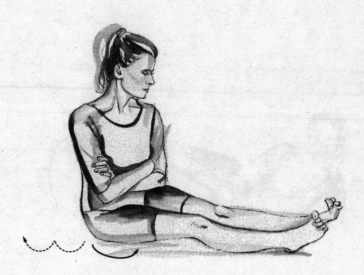

# TO SLIM THE LEGS

1 Lie on your left side, propped up on your left forearm, with your legs together and your right hand on the floor in front of you for support.

2 Raise your right leg and lower it rapidly, ten to twenty times.

3 Repeat on your right side with your left leg.

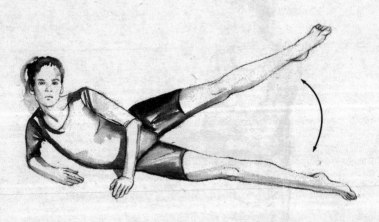

## *TO MAKE YOU MORE FLEXIBLE*

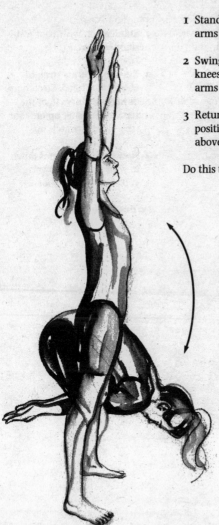

1 Stand with your feet apart, arms stretched overhead.

2 Swing down, with your knees bent, and swing your arms between your legs.

3 Return to the starting position with your arms above your head.

Do this three to five times.

# A SIMPLE STRETCHING EXERCISE FOR THE WHOLE BODY

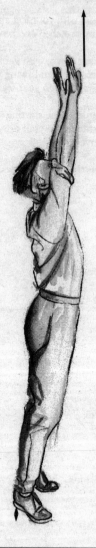

1 Stand erect, with your feet slightly apart.

2 Raise your arms straight above your head. Stretch up as high as you can, at the same time rising up on your toes – really stretch up.

3 Now bring your arms down to your sides and lower your heels to the floor.

Do this three times.

# TO STRETCH THE CALF MUSCLES AND THIGHS

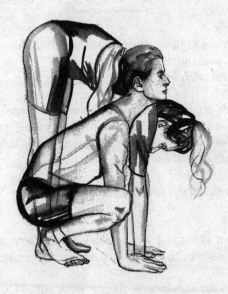

1 Squat with your hands flat on the
   floor in front of you, with your feet
   together, knees apart and heels
   raised.

2 Now straighten your legs, lowering
   your heels while keeping your hands
   on the floor.
   Hold for a count of twenty.

3 Go back to the squatting position.

Do this three times.

# *LOOKING AFTER YOUR HANDS*

The exercises in this section are to help bring more circulation into your arms, hands and fingers. They will prevent the stiffness often felt in the finger joints.

The hands are often said to show the most obvious signs of ageing – and the hands of even fairly young people can appear very aged – but these exercises will help to keep your hands supple and young-looking.

Use a good hand cream if your hands tend to be dry or cracked.

Use cotton gloves for house work when convenient, and certainly wear rubber gloves if using strong detergents.

Massage your hands with slighly moist salt. (The backs of your hands are particularly important.) This will help to remove dead skin and dryness and to keep your hands smooth.

You can do most of these exercises at any time, wherever you happen to be. You need not do them all at the same time – doing individual exercises at odd moments throughout the day is just as good.

# FOR GENERAL LIMBERING UP AND TO PREVENT STIFFNESS

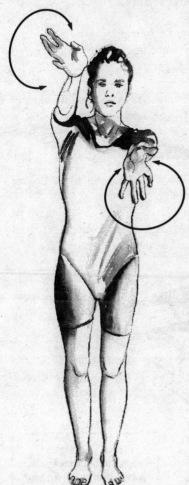

Sit or stand. Look straight ahead.

1 Extend your arms straight out in front of you. Now shake your hands and arms vigorously for a count of ten.

2 Relax with your arms at your sides.

3 Repeat the above, but this time with your arms stretched out to the sides.

Really shake out.

# FOR HAND AND FINGER FLEXIBILITY

Sit, stand or lie down.

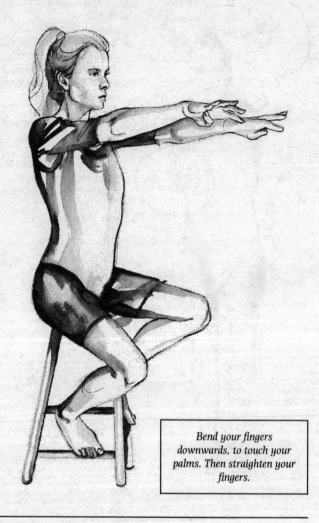

Bend your fingers
downwards, to touch your
palms. Then straighten your
fingers.

## FOR HAND AND FINGER FLEXIBILITY

1 Stretch your arms out in front of you.
   With your palms facing the floor,
   spread your fingers out as far as
   possible.

   Then clench your fingers tightly.

   Do this three times.

   Relax and breathe.

2 Again with your arms stretched out
   in front of you, palms facing the floor,
   try to touch the palms of your hands
   with each of your fingers and your
   thumbs in turn.

   Start with both little fingers, then
   continue with both third fingers and
   so on to both thumbs in turn.

   Do this three times.

   Shake your arms and hands out.

   Relax and breathe.

# FOR GENERAL CIRCULATION AND FLEXIBILITY OF THE JOINTS

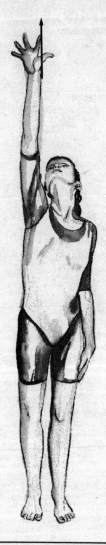

Stand with your feet slightly apart, arms at your sides.

1 Stretch your right arm above your head as far as possible.

2 At the same time, spread your fingers wide apart and look up at your hand. Really stretch up.

3 Now relax with your right arm at your side.

4 Repeat with your left arm.

Do this three times.

> *Have a really good stretch each time.*

# FOR SUPPLENESS OF THE FINGERS AND HANDS

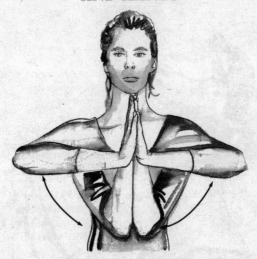

Sit or stand.

1 Rub the palms of your hands together briskly – include your wrists and fingertips.

2 Now press your hands together, fingers facing upwards.

3 Bend your hands at the wrists, keeping your fingers as straight as possible. Fingers should be pointing upwards. Elbows bent out each side.

Hold for a count of five.

Relax and shake out your hands.

If flexible enough, do this three times.

# FOR FLEXIBILITY OF THE FINGERS

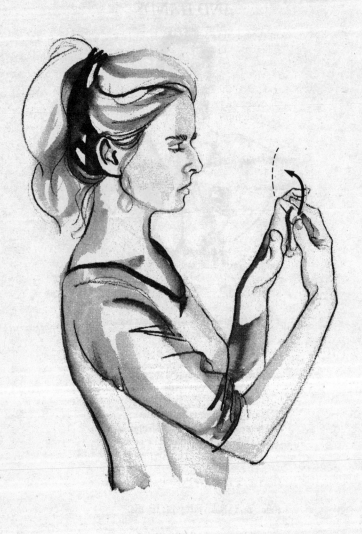

## FOR FLEXIBILITY OF THE FINGERS

In turn, bend each finger at the two
different joints.

1 First at the top joints. Curl each finger
over and press at the top joint, then
straighten (as in the illustration).

2 Then bend in turn each straight finger
towards the palm.

Press gently at the joint.

This exercise helps the energy in the
fingers and joints to flow more freely.

# TO LOOSEN STIFF FINGERS

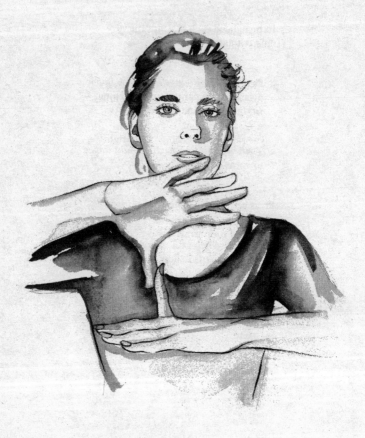

Your fingers may be rather stiff and won't
bend back so far. If so, don't worry and
don't use force.
Your fingers will gradually become more
flexible.

## *TO LOOSEN STIFF FINGERS*

1 Hold one hand in front of you at chest
level, palm down.

2 With the thumb of your other hand,
raise each finger in turn, backwards.

The raised finger should be at right
angles to your hand.

3 Repeat with the other hand.

Shake out your arms, wrists and hands
vigorously.

# A GOOD STRETCHING EXERCISE FOR THE ARMS, HANDS AND FINGERS

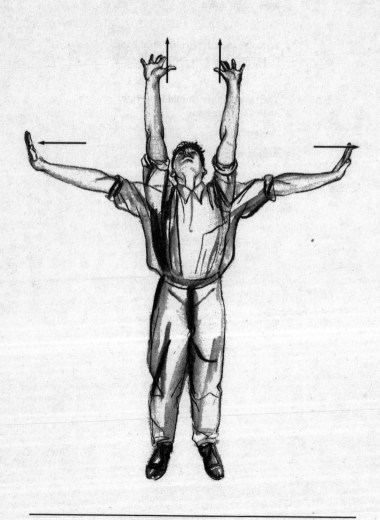

## A GOOD STRETCHING EXERCISE FOR THE ARMS, HANDS AND FINGERS

Stand with your feet slightly apart.

1 Raise your arms above your head, with your palms facing the ceiling.

2 Now, with your fingers spread wide apart, push your palms with all your strength towards the ceiling. Relax with your arms at your sides.

3 Repeat the above exercise but this time with your arms stretched out to the sides, at shoulder level. With your palms facing the side walls, push as hard as you can towards the walls.

Relax with your arms at your sides.

Do the entire exercise three times.

# MASSAGE AND CIRCULATION

Massage is a marvellous way of relaxing tense muscles and getting rid of the tired, drawn expression that these create. By improving the circulation it also gives the complexion a healthy, vibrant glow.

The psychological effects are excellent too – a good massage can replace anxiety, headaches or exhaustion with a feeling of contentment and well-being.

All these benefits mean that including the following massage routines in your overall Workout plan will help you to look and feel years younger.

## BEFORE YOU BEGIN

Start by rubbing your hands together, palm to palm, really briskly up and down for twenty to thirty seconds.

Include the wrists and right up to the fingertips.

Now hold your hands up, with limp wrists, and shake them out from side to side.

Repeat the above from time to time whenever you are touching your face, for added energy.

# TO STIMULATE THE NECK AND LYMPH GLANDS

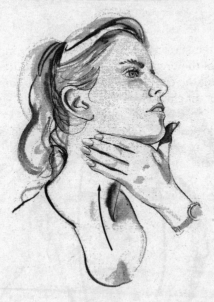

After briskly rubbing your hands together, continue immediately.

Starting with the flat of your hand on your chest, stroke up the front of the neck and under the chin to the jaw line.

Alternate your hands in smooth succession.

Do this ten times with each hand.

# TO HELP THE CIRCULATION IN THE FACE

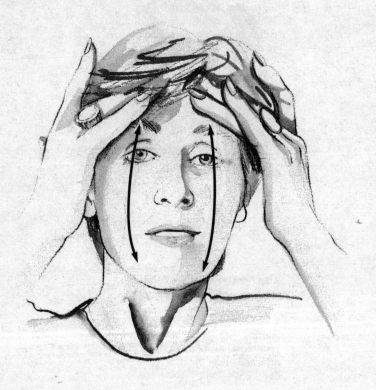

> Remember – use very light, smooth strokes.
> Do not stretch the skin at all.

## TO HELP THE CIRCULATION
## IN THE FACE

After briskly rubbing your hands
together, continue immediately.
With *featherlight* touch, smooth the
palms and fingers of your hands over
your face:

1 Start at the jaw line, then move up
   and over the cheeks and each side of
   the nostrils.

2 Gently smooth over the eyes, and over
   the forehead to the hairline.

3 Continue back down the sides of the
   face to the jaw line.

Do these movements six times in a
continuous motion.

## TO STIMULATE THE EYE AREA

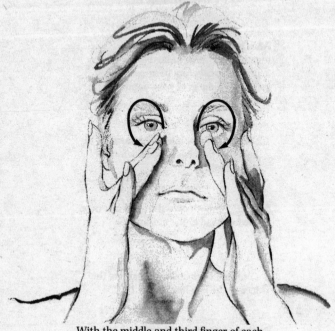

With the middle and third finger of each
hand, smooth around your eye sockets:

1   Start at the bridge of the nose.

2   Smooth outwards along the
    eyebrows.

3   Continue round on to the cheek-bones
    towards the nose.

Make this rotary movement six times.

## TO RELAX THE FOREHEAD

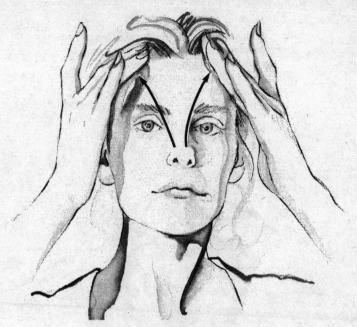

With your fingers, stroke from the bridge
of your nose up and out along your
forehead to your hairline, on each side
of your face.

Do this six times.

# TO RELEASE TENSION IN THE TEMPLES

With your fingertips resting above your temples on each side of your head, use your thumbs to massage the area in front of the ears, from the lobes up to the temples.

Do this three times.

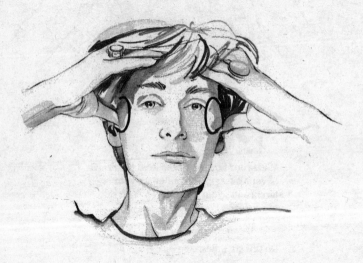

Make small, circular movements.

## *TO STIMULATE THE SCALP*

With the pads of your fingertips,
massage over the entire scalp with small
stationary rotations, for thirty seconds
or more.

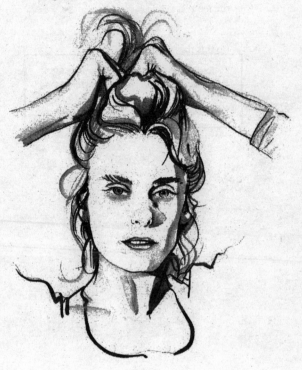

*Take large fistfuls of hair and pull upwards.*
*This stimulates hair growth.*

# TO STIMULATE THE UPPER BODY

With a very flexible wrist, *lightly* pound with your fist on your chest, shoulders, outer side of arms, wrists and backs of hands.

---

*Remember that these exercises are for releasing tension and for gently stimulating your system.*
*Do them whenever you feel a bit tense!*

---

# TO STIMULATE THE UNDER-CHIN AREA

Slap under your chin with the back of
your hand. (One hand will do.) Make
quick, light taps, thirty times.

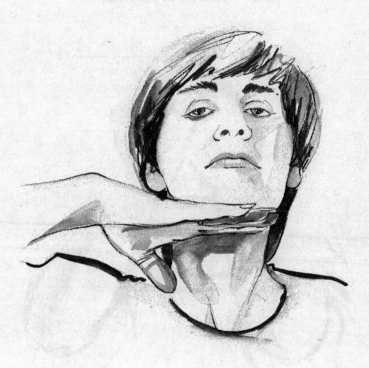

## *PALMING*

Rub your palms together briskly for ten
seconds, then hold them over your eyes
and relax.
Do this whenever you are tired or tense.

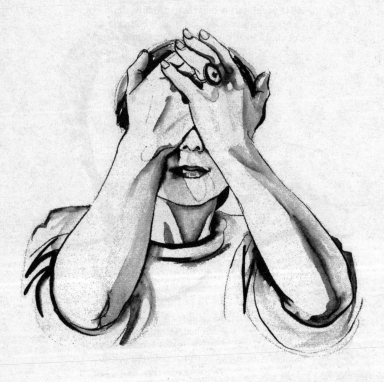

# PRESSURE POINTS FOR THE FACE

In this section and the next, I am going to show you a simple method of stimulating the energy flow to the skin and muscle tissue, bringing further benefit to your Workout programme.

All through our bodies there are tiny channels, known as meridians, through which energy circulates to all our organs, nerves and glands. These life channels can become blocked, slowing down our energy circulation. However, if finger pressure is applied to certain parts of the body, particularly the hands and feet, this life energy will flow freely once more.

Many of you will know this ancient and successful method as reflexology. There are many practitioners and books on this subject if you feel you would like to know more than I shall say about it here.

In this section we are concentrating on the pressure points of the face, ears and neck.

Do the following routine as often as you can – daily, if possible, for the first month, then two or three times a week for maintenance.

You may do this routine sitting, standing or lying down – even in bed, feeling relaxed and warm. To begin with, though, it is better to sit in front of a mirror to learn the different pressure-point positions. This takes no time at all, and afterwards you are free to work out wherever you are.

# PRESSURE POINTS FOR THE FACE

On the illustration, you will see a series of numbers. These are your massage points.

Start at Point 1. Using your middle or index finger, press firmly on the massage point for a count of five.

Now make circular movements on the point, moving upwards then outwards for thirty to forty rotations.

Continue with all the numbered points in turn, up to and including *Point 9*, massaging each point in the same way. Use both hands to massage points on each side of the head where indicated (points 4–8).

*Point 10* With the pads of your thumbs facing towards your ears, stroke down under each cheek-bone until you reach an indentation. This is your point of massage.

*Point 11* See page 158 for ear stimulation.

*Point 12* With the fingers of one hand on one side of your throat and the thumb on the other, massage in quick movements up and down for about twenty rotations. Then change hands and repeat this.

Follow with the tapping routine on page 162.

## PRESSURE POINTS FOR THE FACE

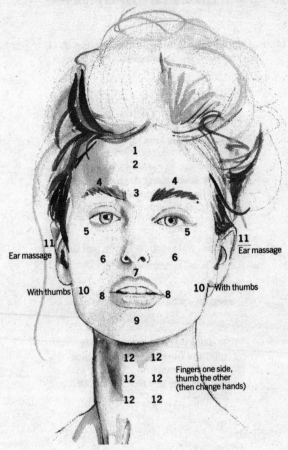

Do not *push your head forward into your
hands.*
*Let your fingers do the work, so relax back.*
*Shake your hands out and breathe freely at
intervals.*

# EAR STIMULATION

This massage is very warming and stimulating. Try it – your face will glow.

1 With your index fingers and thumbs, hold the top rim of your ears and pull upwards. With small rotations, massage this area.

2 Move down along the rim – pull your ears out gently and massage. Continue like this all around the rim.

3 When you reach the lobes, pull the lobes down and again massage.

Repeat this whole exercise once more.

4 Now massage all the crevices or spirals of the ears, with tiny quick circular movements. The pads of the index fingers (*not* the tips) are best for this.

## EAR STIMULATION

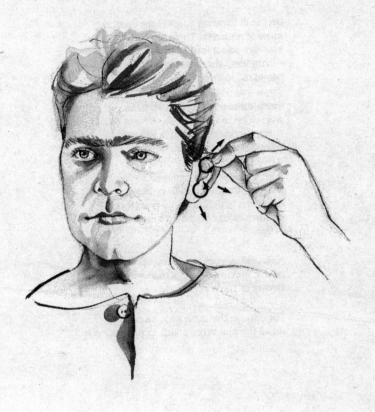

# PRESSURE POINTS FOR THE EYES
# AND NASAL PASSAGES

On the illustration you will see another series of numbers. These are your massage points for the areas surrounding the eyes and nasal passages.

These numbered points need to be worked on to stimulate the flow of energy. In many cases this will help to relieve eye strain and sinus problems.

Start at the points numbered 1.
Use your thumbs, middle or index fingers on both hands and press firmly on the massage points for a count of five.

Now make circular movements on the points, moving upwards then *inwards* for twenty or thirty rotations.

Continue in the same way, massaging on all the numbered points in turn.

---

Do not *push your head forward into your hands.*
*Let your fingers do the work, so relax back.*
*Breathe freely. Feel relaxed.*

## PRESSURE POINTS FOR THE EYES
## AND NASAL PASSAGES

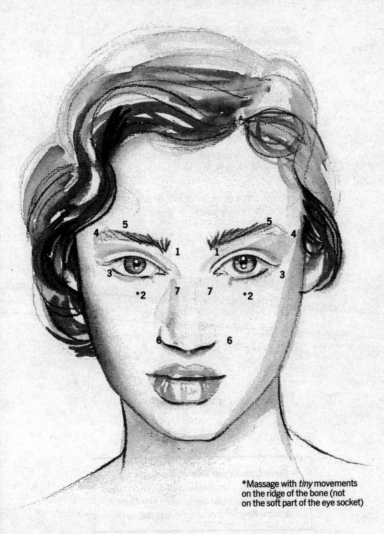

*Massage with *tiny* movements
on the ridge of the bone (not
on the soft part of the eye socket)

# *TAPPING*

Tapping the points shown on the
illustration will help increase circulation.
With the pads of your middle fingers,
tap twenty times at each dot.

Make sharp, light, *very quick* taps (like
testing a very hot iron).

1  Start on your eyebrow (near the
   bridge of your nose). Tap twenty
   times at each point.

2  Repeat this on your cheek-bones (*not*
   in your eye sockets).

3  Work up from your mouth corners,
   ending each side of your nostrils.

4  Work from each side of your chin,
   ending near your ear lobes. Do not
   tap on the jaw bone but slightly
   above, on the fleshy area.

---

*Tapping these points is very quick to do.*
*You can do it any time, anywhere. It is*
*also an excellent routine after you have*
*worked on your pressure points and ears.*

---

## TAPPING POINTS

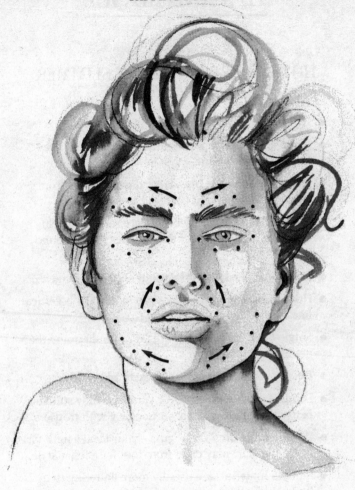

Shake out your hands and shoulders at
intervals, to prevent a build-up of tension.

# TIPS AND ADVICE

## HOW TO DRESS TO LOOK SLIMMER AND YOUNGER

- A trench coat is the most slimming of styles.

- If you are pear-shaped, wearing shoulder pads can improve your outline.

- To counteract wide hips, wear darker shades from the waist down. Light coloured tops are fine.

- Close-fitted tops, tightly belted, are rarely flattering to a large bust. A V neckline is better than a round-necked top.

- V necklines make your face and neck look longer.

- Horizontal stripes will make you look wider – vertical lines are better.

- Single-breasted garments are far more slimming than double-breasted ones.

- Double vents at the back of jackets add width.

- Longish jackets which cover your hips may suit you better than shorter ones, particularly with trousers.

- Experiment with skirt lengths – your ideal length for a straight skirt may differ from that for a fuller style.

- Smooth materials are usually more flattering than fluffy ones, which can seem to add inches to your measurements.

- Shoulders generally look better padded – but not *too* wide.

- Don't wear tight underwear – this can produce bulges under your clothes.

- Full skirts with a smooth yoke over the hips are more slimming than those in which the fullness comes from the waistband.

- Avoid clinging jersey fabrics.

- Trousers with straight, long lines are best – harem styles are not so flattering.

## HAIR

Choose a hairstylist either by recommendation or through a magazine article. *Before* you make an appointment:

- Have a brief consultation with the person who would be cutting your hair and discuss what ideas he or she suggests for you.

- Remember, it is you that has to live with your new haircut – and for quite a while if it is too short – so don't be afraid to say what you like and, importantly, what you dislike.

- Saying 'not too short' is not enough – you must specify the length that you want. However, don't be inflexible but listen to any new ideas – they could be marvellous for you.

- If you lead a busy life you will want an easy-to-manage style. Discuss these aspects.

- Find out the total cost.

If you feel confident in the whole idea, make an appointment. If you don't, try somewhere else.

## COLOUR SENSE

Colour can make an enormous difference to anyone's appearance. If you have an outfit you feel particularly good in, and others say how well you look in it, it is probably not only the shape but also the colour that is working to your advantage.

A simple way to test yourself for colour is first to hold up a black garment in front of you and then try a brown one. Whichever one suits you best determines your basic dark colour. Then do the same with white and cream.

In general terms, if the brown and cream suit you best, you should go more for the autumn shades, with undertones of yellow. For example:

- choose peach (which has a yellow undertone) rather than brighter pinks;

- choose the more yellowy greens, rather than the bluer ones;

- olive should be another suitable choice;

- mustard colours might suit you too.

If the black and white suit you best, choose clearer, more vibrant colours – blues and colours with a bluish undertone. For example:

- choose fuchsia or shocking pink, both of which have a bluish tone, *not* the yellower peach colours;

- choose greens that have a bluish tone, too;

- reds which also have some blue tones should suit you, but certainly nothing too orange, which has added yellow.

These suggestions are, of course, very general and just give you the basic idea. There are many colour consultants around if you want more detailed personal advice.

## SOME FINAL TIPS FOR THE FACE

- For bags under the eyes, in addition to the under-eye exercise on page 53, lie on the floor and place two cold used tea-bags – partly squeezed out – over your closed eyes. Relax like this for ten to twenty minutes.

- When relaxing, take yourself in your mind to a peaceful place you would enjoy – the beach, the mountains, the countryside – anywhere that gives you pleasure.

- Don't put moisturizer on the area surrounding your eyes.

- For a longer neck and a better jaw line, sit up straight. Imagine you are being lifted up by the hair on the crown of your head.